The Role of Drug Treatments for Eating Disorders

BRUNNER/MAZEL
EATING DISORDERS MONOGRAPH SERIES

Series Editors
Paul E. Garfinkel, M.D.
David M. Garner, Ph.D.

The Role of Drug Treatments for Eating Disorders

Edited by

PAUL E. GARFINKEL, M.D.
Professor of Psychiatry, University of Toronto;
Psychiatrist-in-Chief, Toronto General Hospital

and

DAVID M. GARNER, Ph.D.
Professor of Psychiatry, University of Toronto;
Research Director, Division of Psychiatry, Toronto General Hospital

BRUNNER/MAZEL, *Publishers* • New York

Library of Congress Cataloging-in-Publication Data

The Role of drug treatments for eating disorders.

Includes bibliographies and index.
1. Appetite disorders—Chemotherapy.
2. Psychotropic drugs. I. Garfinkel, Paul E.,
1946-   . II. Garner, David M., 1947-   .
[DNLM: 1. Anorexia Nervosa—drug therapy. 2. Bulimia—
drug therapy. WM 175 R745]
RC552.E18R65   1987   616.85′2   86-33367
ISBN 0-87630-460-9

Copyright © 1987 by Paul E. Garfinkel and David M. Garner

Published by
BRUNNER/MAZEL, INC.
19 Union Square
New York, New York 10003

All rights reserved. No part of this book may be reproduced
by any process whatsoever without the written permission of the copyright owners.

MANUFACTURED IN THE UNITED STATES OF AMERICA

Contents

Contributors vii
Introduction xi

1. Drug Therapies for Eating Disorders:
   Monoamine Oxidase Inhibitors 3
   Sidney Kennedy and B. Timothy Walsh

2. Use of Tricyclic Antidepressants in Anorexia Nervosa
   and Bulimia Nervosa 36
   David B. Herzog and Andrew W. Brotman

3. Uses and Potential Misuses of Antianxiety Agents in
   the Treatment of Anorexia Nervosa and
   Bulimia Nervosa 59
   Arnold E. Andersen

4. The Use of Neuroleptics in the Treatment of
   Anorexia Nervosa Patients 74
   Walter Vandereycken

5. Lithium in the Treatment of Eating Disorders ... 90
   L. K. George Hsu

6. Anticonvulsant Treatment of Eating Disorders ... 96
   Allan S. Kaplan

7. Serotonin in Eating Disorders: Theory and Therapy ... 124
   David S. Goldbloom

8. Opioid Antagonist Drugs in the Treatment of
   Anorexia Nervosa 150
   Walter H. Kaye

9. Drugs That Facilitate Gastric Emptying 161
   *Gerry Craigen, Sidney Kennedy, Paul E. Garfinkel,
   and Khursheed Jeejeebhoy*

Name Index 181
Subject Index 189

Contributors

Arnold E. Andersen, M.D.
Associate Professor, Psychiatry and Behavioral Sciences,
The Johns Hopkins University School of Medicine,
The Johns Hopkins Hospital, Baltimore, Maryland.

Andrew W. Brotman, M.D.
Supervisor, Eating Disorders Unit and Chief, Freedom
Trail Clinic, Eric Lindemann Mental Health; and Assistant
Professor of Psychiatry, Massachusetts General Hospital,
Harvard Medical School.

Gerry Craigen, M.D.
Chief Resident in Psychiatry, Toronto General Hospital,
University of Toronto.

David S. Goldbloom, M.D., F.R.C.P. (C)
Centennial Fellow, Medical Research Council of Canada;
Lecturer, Department of Psychiatry, University of
Toronto; and Psychiatrist, Toronto General Hospital.

David B. Herzog, M.D.
Director, Eating Disorders Unit, Massachusetts General
Hospital; and Assistant Professor of Psychiatry, Harvard
Medical School.

L. K. George Hsu, M.D.
Associate Professor of Psychiatry; and
Director, Outpatient Eating Disorders Program,
University of Pittsburgh School of Medicine,
Western Psychiatric Institute and Clinic,
Pittsburgh, Pennsylvania.

Khursheed Jeejeebhoy, M.B.
Head, Division of Gastroenterology, Toronto General
Hospital; and Professor of Medicine, University of
Toronto.

Allan S. Kaplan, M.D., F.R.C.P.(C)
Medical Director, Eating Disorders Center, Toronto
General Hospital; and Assistant Professor of Psychiatry,
University of Toronto.

Walter H. Kaye, M.D.
Associate Professor and Program Director, Inpatient
Eating Disorders Program, University of Pittsburgh
School of Medicine, Department of Psychiatry, Western
Psychiatric Institute and Clinic, Pittsburgh, Pennsylvania.

Sidney Kennedy, M.B.
Head, Nutritional and Affective Disorders Service,
Toronto General Hospital; and Assistant Professor,
University of Toronto.

Walter Vandereycken, M.D., Ph.D. Med. Sci.
Associate Professor of Psychopathology, University of
Leuven, Belgium; and Head of the Anorexia Nervosa
Unit, University Psychiatric Center, Kortenberg,
Belgium.

B. Timothy Walsh, M.D.
Associate Professor of Clinical Psychiatry, Department of Psychiatry, Columbia University College of Physicians and Surgeons; and the New York State Psychiatric Institute, New York, New York.

Introduction

Anorexia nervosa and bulimia nervosa are receiving increasing attention in the scientific literature for a number of reasons: (1) They have increased dramatically in frequency since 1970 and are now commonly encountered in clinical practice; (2) today anorexia nervosa and bulimia nervosa are associated with a significant mortality—between 5% and 10% of patients die; and (3) a chronic form of the illness develops in about 25% of patients. The latter includes a group of people who are chronically at low body weight or display wide fluctuations in body weight with regular purging and its complications, including hypokalemia. Frequently, there are psychosocial sequelae including a high prevalence of anxiety and affective disorders and markedly isolated lifestyles. The significant mortality and the morbidity and prevalence of these disorders have justified the tremendous increase in research devoted to their understanding and better treatment.

Much has been learned in the past 15 years about the diagnosis and understanding of people who have such serious eating disorders. Especially important has been the acceptance of a model of understanding these disorders based on multiple risk factors—a biopsychosocial model as described by Weiner and Engel for illness in general. Such a model implies not only a variety of risk factors for a particular disorder but also that a disorder may be perpetuated by factors very different from those which have produced it. This type of model also implies the need for multiple aspects to treatment both within and across individuals. Although this generally means that the clinician must pay attention to various factors that have perpetuated the illness as well as risk factors, this does not mean anything or everything is acceptable in treatment. Certain basic principles have come to be recognized to be the cornerstones of treatment by most people who specialize in this area regardless of their particular theoretical orientation.

The basic principles of treatment now include: (1) the need for weight restoration so that the effects of starvation on a person's thinking, feeling, and behavior may be minimized and so that she may face her phobia of her normal body size; and (2) the need for an ongoing psychotherapy to enable the individual to work through factors that have contributed to the chronicity and also placed her at risk initially. Use of this model has permitted more widespread acceptance of the need for different approaches to treatment for different aspects of the patients' problems. What is useful for helping someone regain weight may be very different from helping the patient to adjust to a particular marital or work situation or a chronic depressive disorder.

Drug therapies are of some interest and are the particular subject matter of this volume. Clinicians have approached the use of drug therapies for eating disorders for very different reasons.

1. Drug therapies may be selected based on a practitioner's conceptualization of the nature of the eating disorder. For example, if excess cortisol secretion is considered to be the primary problem in anorexia nervosa, it is understandable that the practitioner would orient treatment to reducing cortisol levels. This example is current since such treatments are now being advocated for treating anorexia nervosa, in spite of the fact that there is no support from the experimental literature to suggest that these cortisol changes either are of primary significance or are causative for any of the symptom clusters that develop. Similarly, if one views that bulimia nervosa is the result of neurophysiological dysregulation in the hypothalamus, the use of anticonvulsant medication becomes logical. If the eating disorders are viewed as atypical or unusual manifestations of an affective illness, the use of tricyclic antidepressants or MAOI becomes logical.

2. Others may begin to explore and recommend the use of

medications not because of their theoretical approach to the nature of the disorder, but rather because of observable symptom clusters which occur in these patients and which may be amenable to pharmacotherapy as adjuncts to an overall treatment program involving nutritional support, education, and psychotherapy. It is from this latter perspective that the current volume has originated. Clinicians and investigators are beginning to recognize the need for using medication for selected individuals based on the presence of certain symptom clusters without it implying a primary cause of the illness. It is assumed from this point of view that because one patient with an eating disorder has benefited from medication does not mean that such medicine should be used routinely for all such patients.

The primary aims of this book are to provide the clinician with a guide for the use of medication as a possible adjunct to an overall treatment program, to provide an element of caution by highlighting when medication is not indicated, and to outline possible areas for further research that may enrich treatment in the future. Again it must be emphasized that the contributors to this volume do not recommend treatment entirely from a pharmacological point of view. In some of the areas covered, little research has been done at present; however, it may be anticipated that significant advances will be made in the future by a better understanding of pharmacologic treatments. For example, little work has been done on serotonin reuptake inhibitors, but based on the biological changes that occur in starvation and in the brain in serotonin metabolism it makes good sense to explore further the possible use of drugs such as Tryptophan and Fluoxetine.

Some cautionary notes are required:

1. This volume does not provide a detailed discussion of the psychology or psychosocial treatments for eating disorders not because these are viewed to be unimportant but rather because they have been considered in some detail elsewhere (Garfinkel & Garner, 1982; Garner & Garfinkel, 1985).

2. As is often the case within a relatively new field, in medicine, there is a lack of well-designed and well-described research upon which the clinician may base his or her clinical decisions. There have been significant improvements in this regard in the literature on eating disorders in the last five years. Information in each area described is at present limited; however small and flawed, we did feel that it was important to provide a synthesis of the existing literature at this time.

3. Studies thus far have not properly compared pharmacotherapies with other therapeutic modalities or their combinations. It is not possible, therefore, to offer definitive comments about such comparisons or whether the effectiveness of treatments is truly additive, as, for example, studies on depression have shown.

4. There is some evidence to date for the efficacy of medication in some patients with bulimia nervosa: for example, MAOI and tricyclic antidepressants. But this does not mean that these medications should be applied routinely for all patients. Rather we must search for predictive factors to determine who will respond to these medications. In each chapter an investigator/clinician who has demonstrated a special expertise with a particular pharmacologic approach describes what is currently known about that approach.

5. Care must be taken regarding side effects. Although clinicians constantly weigh the benefits versus the risks of any treatment modality for every patient, this is especially important for those patients who are physically ill, as are so many who suffer from eating disorders. There may be some theoretical benefit to a medication for some patients, yet they may not be able to tolerate these medicines because of side effects. Other risks may develop over a longer period of time that may prevent the long-term use of medication. For example, the initial literature on the use of MAOIs in bulimia nervosa appears promising, yet these patients seem to experience many side effects that preclude their long-term use of the medication.

6. It is an error to assume that we understand the pathophysiology of a disorder based on patients' responsiveness to a particular

medication and knowledge of how that medication works. All psychotropic medications affect multiple systems, and benefits for one group of patients may be the result of one set of properties of the medicine, whereas patients with other problems may benefit from the medication's effects on other systems.

Finally, bringing together this information has highlighted a number of unanswered questions for future research. We are hopeful that when this subject is reviewed, at a later date, there will be a noticeable improvement in the amount of information available and how this information is translated into benefits to our patients.

September, 1986   PAUL E. GARFINKEL, M.D.
                    DAVID M. GARNER, Ph.D.

REFERENCES

Garfinkel, P. E., & Garner, D. M. *Anorexia Nervosa: A Multidimensional Perspective.* New York: Brunner/Mazel, 1982.

Garner, D. M., & Garfinkel, P. E. (Eds.). *Handbook of Psychotherapy for Anorexia Nervosa and Bulimia.* New York: Guilford Press, 1985.

The Role of Drug Treatments for Eating Disorders

1

Drug Therapies for Eating Disorders: Monoamine Oxidase Inhibitors

Sidney Kennedy and B. Timothy Walsh

In this chapter we examine two topics of relevance to the pharmacological approach to treatment of eating disorders. First, because there has long been an interest in the treatment of anorexia nervosa and, more recently, of bulimia nervosa with antidepressant agents, we discuss the relationship between eating disorders and disturbances of mood. Second, we review the information currently available on the utility of one specific class of antidepressants—the monoamine oxidase inhibitors (MAOIs)—in the treatment of eating disorders.

THE RELATIONSHIP BETWEEN EATING DISORDERS AND AFFECTIVE ILLNESS

The occurrence of mood disturbances among patients with anorexia nervosa and bulimia nervosa is a facet of both of these syn-

---

We gratefully acknowledge the assistance of Carrol Whynot and Brenda Lediett in Toronto and Evelyn Baronian in New York.

This work was also supported by the Canadian Psychiatric Research Foundation (Dr. S. Kennedy).

dromes that has prompted attempts at pharmacological treatment. The most extreme hypothesis is that eating disorders are variants of typical depressive illness, and therefore strategies that are effective for the treatment of depressed patients will be effective for the treatment of patients with eating disorders. In this section we will review information pertinent to the relationship between mood disturbances and eating disorders.

A. Phenomenology

There is broad agreement that, at least in descriptive terms, many patients with eating disorders have disturbances of mood. A number of experienced clinicians have commented on the presence of depression in patients with anorexia nervosa and structured measures of depression have documented this impression (Bruch, 1973; Folstein, Wakeling, & De Souza, 1977; Halmi, Goldberg, Eckert, Casper, & Davis, 1977; Piran, Kennedy, Garfinkel, & Owens, 1985). There have been surprisingly few studies of the frequency of depressive syndromes among patients with anorexia nervosa, perhaps, in part, because of the difficulty of assessing mood in the face of starvation. Still, the few studies that have used structured diagnostic interviews in anorexia nervosa have found a prevalence of depressive syndromes that were higher than expected among controls (Biederman, Rivinus, Herzog, Ferber, & Harper et al., 1984; Piran et al., 1985; Strober, 1982).

A second indication of a link between anorexia nervosa and mood disturbances is derived from follow-up studies of patients with anorexia nervosa. These studies have generally noted a significant prevalence of mood disturbance among patients once treated for anorexia nervosa, and a high frequency of suicides (Cantwell, Sturzenberger, Burroughs, Salkin, & Green, 1977; Hsu, 1980; Theander, 1970). From the data currently available, it is unclear to what degree depression on follow-up is related to the persistence and severity of the eating disorder. However, the mere presence of a significant depression in these follow-up studies suggests that there is *some* relationship between anorexia nervosa and depression.

A phenomenologic association between depression and bulimia nervosa in normal-weight individuals has also been described. Russell, in his original description of the syndrome of bulimia nervosa (1979), noted that "next to the preoccupations directly concerned with eating and weight, depressive symptoms were the most prominent feature of the patients' mental state." Subsequent authors have generally concurred with this view. Fairburn and Cooper (1984) using the Present State Examination, Weiss and Ebert (1983) using the SCL-90, Johnson and Larson (1982) using an analogue rating scale, and Abraham and Beumont (1982) using a structured clinical interview have all noted a high frequency of depressed mood and of symptoms of anxiety. In addition to these descriptive studies, several investigators have attempted to determine how many patients with bulimia nervosa meet the criteria for syndromes of disturbed mood. The frequencies of current major depressive illness using structured interview schedules range from 20% to 70% (Herzog, 1984; Hudson, Pope, Jonas, & Yurgelun-Todd, 1983b; Piran et al., 1985; Walsh, Roose, Glassman, Gladis, & Sadik, 1985b) and lifetime frequencies for major depression appear to be over 50%. The depressive syndrome, when it occurs, is rarely of an endogenous or melancholic type, but rather appears to be characterized by a reactive mood and a significant degree of anxiety. Most descriptions of patients with bulimia nervosa highlight the presence of anxiety. In fact, in the reports of Hudson, Pope, and Jonas (1983a), and of Piran et al. (1985), about one-half of the patients with bulimia nervosa met DSM-III criteria for panic disorder.

B. Family History

One of the striking characteristics of serious mood disturbances is their tendency to run in families. An increased frequency of mood disturbance among the relatives of patients with eating disorders would provide convincing evidence of some type of relationship between these two illnesses. Several studies have reviewed the frequency of psychiatric illness among the relatives of patients with anorexia nervosa (Cantwell et al., 1977; Gershon, Hamovit, Schreiber et al., 1983; Hudson et al., 1983b; Piran et al., 1985; Rivinus, Biederman, Herzog, Kemper & Harper, et al., 1984; Strober, Salkin, Burroughs, & Morrell, 1982; Theander, 1970; Winokur, March, & Mendels, et al., 1980), and all have found an increased frequency of depressive illness. These data are among the most convincing evidence of a link between anorexia nervosa and major depressive illness. These data do not, however, prove that there is a genetic link between depressive illness and anorexia nervosa, since growing up in a family environment with significant depressive illness may increase one's vulnerability to develop anorexia nervosa. In addition, because of the high prevalence of mood disturbance among patients with anorexia nervosa, the implications of increased familial frequencies of affective disorders are unclear. That is, it is currently uncertain whether the increased family history of mood disorders rests primarily on data from families of patients who themselves are depressed or whether there is an increased frequency of mood disorders even among the relatives of patients who do not have mood disturbances (Biederman, Rivinus, Kemper, Hamilton, & MacFayden, et al., 1985b; Gershon, Schreiber, Hamovit, Dibble, & Kaye, et al., 1984).

Several uncontrolled studies have noted what appeared to be an increased frequency of depression among the families of patients of normal body weight with bulimia nervosa (Fairburn & Cooper, 1984; Pyle, Mitchell, & Eckert, 1981). Two controlled studies have attempted to evaluate the frequency of mood disturbance among the relatives of patients of normal body weight with bulimia nervosa and have compared these to the frequencies of relatives of control subjects. Hudson et al. (1983b) found an increased frequency of depressive diagnoses among the relatives of bulimic patients compared to the relatives of patients with schizophrenia or with borderline personality disorder. However, Stern and co-workers (1984) were unable to document increased familial frequency of depression in bulimic individuals compared to normal controls. The latter study included in its control group several individuals with known mood disturbance and may therefore have elevated the control frequency of familial mood disturbance. Thus, at present, although there are hints of an increased frequency of mood disturbance in the families of patients with bulimia nervosa, this issue is not settled. The prevalence of eating disorders in the families of affective-disorder patients has also not yet been definitively reported.

C. Biological Measures

There has been great excitement in the last decade concerning the utility of biological measures in the diagnosis of major mood disturbance. The two parameters that have probably received the greatest attention are the activity of the hypothalamic-pituitary-adrenal axis and the nature of sleep in patients with major depression.

There is now little doubt that a significant number, approximately 50%, of patients with "endogenous" depression secrete greater amounts of the adrenal hormone cortisol than do normal subjects. This phenomenon has been documented by a number of investigators using a variety of techniques including indwelling catheters in which cortisol concentration in the blood is measured over a 24-hour period (Sachar, Hellman, Roffwarg, Halpern, & Fukushima, et al., 1973). A substantial fraction of patients with endogenous depression also show disturbances of cortisol suppression following the administration of dexamethasone, and it has been suggested that this disturbance may be utilized in the diagnosis of depressive illness (Carroll, Feinberg, Greden, Tarika, & Albala, et al., 1981).

It is clear that a number of abnormalities of the hypothalamic-pituitary-adrenal axis occur in anorexia nervosa and that, in some ways, these disturbances resemble those found in major depression.

Specifically, patients with anorexia nervosa typically exhibit elevated levels of plasma cortisol and abnormal cortisol responses to dexamethasone suppression at low weight similar to those of patients with major depression (Boyar, Hellman, Roffwarg, Katz, & Zumoff, et al., 1977). Yet, similar disturbances also occur in any form of malnutrition, and in most anorexic subjects weight restoration alone results in the normalization of cortisol secretory patterns (Kennedy, Stokl, Garfinkel, Wilkes, & Stern-Mighton, et al., 1984; Walsh, 1982). Thus, although there are similarities between the adrenal axis disturbances of anorexia nervosa and depression, this does not necessarily imply that patients with anorexia nervosa have a similar psychobiological illness.

Several studies of normal-weight patients with bulimia nervosa have found a higher than expected frequency of nonsuppression to the dexamethasone suppression test (Gwirtsman, Roy-Byrne, Yager, & Gerner, 1983; Hudson et al., 1983a; Lindy, Walsh, Roose, Gladis, Glassman, 1985). These findings have been interpreted as indicating that a significant fraction of patients of normal body weight with bulimia nervosa show increases in hypothalamic-pituitary-adrenal activity similar to that found in patients with endogenous depression.

However, there are some difficulties associated with this conclusion. First, it has become clear that abnormalities of the dexamethasone suppression test are not specific to major depressive illness. Patients with a variety of other psychiatric diagnoses, including dementia, mania, and acute psychosis, have been reported as having abnormal responses to the dexamethasone suppression test. Second, whereas several groups have reported abnormalities of the DST in bulimia nervosa, no group has yet established an abnormality of the basal secretion of cortisol. Walsh and colleagues (1986) have found that the 24-hour plasma concentration of cortisol in 12 patients of normal weight with bulimia nervosa was normal. Calabrese and co-workers (1985) have recently reported that the basal cortisol level and the cortisol response to the hypothalamic hormone corticotropin releasing factor (CRF) were also normal in normal weight patients with bulimia nervosa. These data suggest that, although the dexamethasone suppression test may be abnormal, the hypothalamic-pituitary-adrenal axis does not appear to be hyperactive in most patients of normal weight with bulimia nervosa. Further studies of the HPA axis in this syndrome are required to elucidate this paradox but, at this point it seems premature to conclude that patients of normal weight with bulimia nervosa have disturbances described in patients with endogenous depression. Similar limitations apply to the interpretation of other shared endocrine abnormalities such as those within the thyroid axis.

It is now relatively well established that major depressive illness is associated with abnormalities of sleep monitored by EEG, including shortened REM latency, increased REM density, and reduced slow wave sleep (Coble, Foster, & Kupfer, 1976; Gillin, Duncan, Pettigrew, Frankel, & Snyder, 1979). Many underweight patients with anorexia nervosa complain of sleep disturbances, and a few patients with anorexia nervosa have been described as having REM latencies that are well below the normal range (Katz, Kuperberg, Pollack, Walsh, & Zumoff, et al., 1984; Walsh, Goetz, Roose, Fingeroth, & Glassman, 1985a). However, the EEG-monitored characteristics of the sleep of most patients with anorexia nervosa do not appear to resemble those of typical depressive illness.

Three groups have presented data on EEG sleep measures in patients with bulimia nervosa. Walsh et al. (1985a) reported that the sleep of 12 patients with bulimia nervosa was not distinguishable from that of nine control subjects, although the sleep measures may have been distorted by the presence of an intravenous catheter for simultaneous neuroendocrine studies. Levy and colleagues (1985) also failed to separate anorexic, bulimic, and control subjects on the basis of REM latency, whereas Hudson and associates (1985a) reported that normal weight patients with bulimia nervosa had shortened REM latencies compared to normal controls. This would be consistent with the hypothesis that patients with bulimia nervosa have sleep abnormalities similar to those of patients with depression. Thus, although there are some hints of similar disturbances of sleep in eating disorders and depression, it not yet clear how many patients with eating disorders have EEG-monitored sleep disturbances similar to those described in endogenous depression.

In summary, there is broad agreement among investigators working with patients with eating disorders that such patients are prone to have disturbances of mood. However, it is much less clear what relationship the syndromes of anorexia nervosa and bulimia nervosa have to major affective illness. At one extreme it can be argued that the mood disturbances are simply secondary to a serious eating disorder. With regard to anorexia nervosa, this argument may be particularly relevant as there is good evidence that starvation imposed by external circumstances is associated with mood disturbance (Keys, Brozek, Henschel, Mickelsen, & Taylor, 1950). At the other extreme, eating disorders can be viewed as atypical manifestations of depressive illness. It is widely appreciated that disturbances of weight and appetite are prominent in depressive illness, and the salient feature of bulimia nervosa, overeating, has been noted as a symptom of atypical depression (Klein, Gittelman, Quitkin, & Rifkin, 1980). Between these two extremes are a wide variety of other possible relationships between eating disorders and major affective illness. It is currently quite unclear which possibility best explains the association between these syndromes.

THE CLINICAL USE OF MAO INHIBITORS

MAO inhibitors (MAOIs) were first reported to have antidepressant effects over 30 years ago, but their role in psychopharmacology, even today, remains controversial. The decline in their usage in the 1960s, particularly in the United States, was related initially to reports of hypertensive crises when foods with significant tyramine content or stimulant drugs were concomitantly consumed. This "cheese reaction" was felt to occur more often with tranylcypromine which was temporarily withdrawn in the United States. However, when Pare (1985) surveyed the reported tranylcypromine-related deaths in the United Kingdom between 1975 and 1983, he found seven. This represents one death per 14,000 patient years; a figure well below the mortality rate from depression. Much more problematic are the frequent nonfood or drug-related side effects, which are discussed later.

The second "blow" for the MAOIs came from the widely quoted British Medical Research Council collaborative study (Medical Research Council, 1965) comparing ECT, imipramine, and phenelzine in which it was concluded that phenelzine was no more effective than placebo. With such a reputation for potential harm and ineffectiveness, it is perhaps surprising that this group of drugs survived on the pharmacological marketplace. Critics of this trial pointed out that phenelzine was inadequately studied—only hospitalized patients were involved, the dosage was too low, and the duration of the study was too short.

Renewed interest in the MAOIs has been prompted by more rigorous research studies that have been conducted since 1970 which permit two major questions to be addressed: (1) Has efficacy been established in any psychiatric population? (2) Is there a therapeutic advantage of MAOIs over other pharmacotherapies either in general or in a specific subgroup of patients?

1. Clinical Efficacy—MAO Inhibitor Versus Placebo

(a) Affective disorders

Table 1-1 outlines the placebo-controlled double-blind studies published since 1970. These studies have convincingly demonstrated antidepressant effect for MAOIs compared to placebo. Most studies have involved phenelzine, with average dosages of 60–75 mg for at least six weeks. Clinical trials using doses of 40–60 mg of isocarboxazid also showed a good antidepressant effect (Davidson & Turnbull, 1983; Davidson, Weiss, Sullivan, Turnbull, & Linnoila, 1981; Giller, Bialos, Riddle, & Sholomskas, 1982; Zisook, 1983). Earlier studies of tranylcypromine (Glick, 1964; Khanna, Pratt, & Burdizk, 1963) lacked methodological rigor. More recently, Him-

Table 1-1

MAOI-Placebo-Controlled Studies in Depression and Anxiety

Source	Patient Description	Dosage (mg/day)	Duration (wks)	Outcome
Phenelzine-Placebo Studies				
Robinson et al. (1973)	outpatients with primary depressive illness or illness secondary to preexisting anxiety or phobic disorder	60	6	phenelzine (PH) superior to placebo-features of atypical depression showed particularly good improvement
Johnstone & Marsh (1973)	outpatients with neurotic depression	45–90	3	patients receiving PH showed more improvement than those receiving placebo
Tyrer et al. (1973)	patients with agoraphobia	45–90	8	overall assessment of patients on PH significantly improved compared to patients on placebo
Solyom et al. (1973)	phobic patients	45	12	significantly greater overall improvement in patients receiving PH compared to those receiving placebo
Raskin et al. (1974)	neurotic depressives	45	4–7	patients receiving PH did not improve significantly compared to patients receiving placebo; but high dropout rate and relatively low dose of PH
Ravaris et al. (1976)	patients similar to those in Robinson (1973) study	30 & 60	6	patients receiving 60 mg/day PH did significantly better than those receiving 30 mg/day PH who did no better than those receiving placebo

Table 1-1 (*continued*)

Source	Patient Description	Dosage (mg/day)	Duration (wks)	Outcome
Phenelzine-Placebo Studies (*continued*)				
Mountjoy et al. (1977)	anxious patients, depressed patients, and patients with phobic neuroses	45–70	3	overall, patients on PH showed significant improvement compared to placebo; but anxious neurotics had a significant increase in anxiety
Isocarboxazid-Placebo Studies				
Giller et al. (1982)	outpatients meeting DSM-III criteria for major depressive disorder, also having dysphoric mood and anxiety	40–80	6	isocarboxazid (ISO) significantly superior to placebo-trends suggesting anxiety improved first, followed by depression, and then cognitive outlook
Davidson & Turnbull (1983)	outpatients with major or minor depression secondary to generalized or phobic anxiety	10–70	6	patients receiving ISO had greater improvement than those receiving placebo—those with atypical depression responded better than those with typical depression
Zisook (1983)	outpatients with nonpsychotic, nonmelancholic, anxious depression	20–80	6	patients receiving ISO showed significantly more improvement than those receiving placebo
Zisook et al. (1985)	outpatients with atypical depression	20–80	6	overall, patients receiving ISO showed greater improvement than those receiving placebo

(*continued*)

Table 1-1 (*continued*)

Source	Patient Description	Dosage (mg/day)	Duration (wks)	Outcome
Tranylcypromine-Placebo Studies				
Himmelhoch et al. (1982)	outpatients with primary or secondary major affective disorder and anergia	10– ?	6	patients receiving tranylcypromine (TR) showed significantly more improvement than those receiving placebo

melhoch and colleagues (1982) reported rapid and effective response to tranylcypromine at unspecified doses.

(b) Anxiety-related disorders

There is similar agreement that MAOIs are effective anxiolytic agents (Kelly, Guirguis, Frommer, Mitchell-Heggs, & Sargant, 1970; Nies & Robinson, 1981; Solyom, Heseltine, McClure, Solyom, & Lewidge, et al., 1973; Tyrer, Candy, & Kelly, 1973). This effect does not appear to be dependent on concomitant depressive symptoms (Pohl, Berchou, & Rainey, 1982). Phenelzine has also been shown to reduce anticipatory anxiety and to have antiphobic effects (Sheehan, Ballenger, & Jacobsen, 1980).

In the study of Tyrer and colleagues (1980), patients were divided into three diagnostic groups: depressive neurosis, anxiety neurosis, and phobic anxiety. Although those who received the higher dose of phenelzine (90mg) responded significantly better than those on low-dose phenelzine (45mg), there was no difference in quality or rate of response between the three diagnostic groups. Tyrer concluded that phenelzine did not appear to be primarily anxiolytic, antidepressant, or antiphobic in its action and proposed that it acted more as a delayed psychostimulant.

2. Selective Efficacy—MAO Inhibitors Versus Tricyclic Antidepressants (Table 1-2)

There is a commonly held view that patients who respond to tricyclic antidepressants differ from those who respond to MAOIs. This concept is based on reports such as that by Hamilton (1974) that response to ECT was different in patients who failed to respond to phenelzine compared to those who failed to respond to imipramine.

In earlier reports of "atypical depression," West and Dally (1959) and Sargant (1961) noted that MAOI responders often had symptoms of "atypical depression" including hysterical features, phobias, prominent anxiety, and lack of "endogenous" symptoms. Klein and associates (Klein & Davis, 1968; Liebowitz & Klein, 1979; Liebowitz, Quitkin, Stewart, McGrath, & Harrison, et al., 1984) used the term *hysteroid dysphoria* to describe a MAOI responsive syndrome characterized by histrionic personality, high activity and energy when not depressed, rejection sensitivity, symptoms of overeating, oversleeping, and extreme fatigue, and a labile mood that responds temporarily to praise or attention. Although the existence of this syndrome is controversial (Spitzer & Williams, 1982), several recent studies (Kayser, Robinson, Nies, & Howard, 1985; Liebowitz et al., 1984) have continued to report an advantage for phenelzine over imipramine and amitriptyline respectively, in patients with "hysteroid dysphoria."

However, other comparisons between MAOIs and tricyclics (Ravaris, Robinson, Ives, Nies, & Bartlett, 1980; Rowan, Paykel, & Parker, 1982; Sheehan et al., 1980) have shown only minor differences. For example, Rowan and colleagues found only a weak tendency for better response to phenelzine than amitriptyline in patients receiving additional diagnoses of anxiety neurosis.

Finally, although it has generally been stated that MAOIs are less effective in severely "endogenously" depressed inpatients, phenelzine has usually been the comparative agent. More recently Murphy and colleagues (1984a) have suggested that differential biochemical

Table 1-2
MAOI-Tricyclic-Controlled Studies in Depression and Anxiety

Source	Patient Description	MAOI Dosage (Phenelzine) (mg/day)	Comparison Drug	TCA Dosage (mg/day)	Duration (wks)	Outcome
Phenelzine Studies						
Ballenger et al. (1977)	agoraphobics with panic attacks	45–60	imipramine and placebo	150–200	12	phenelzine (PH) and imipramine (IMI) superior to placebo; nonsignificant trend for PH over IMI
Ravaris et al. (1980)	depressed, anxious outpatients	60	amitriptyline	150	6	PH and amitriptyline (AMI) patients show similar overall improvement with PH showing greater antianxiety effects
Sheehan et al. (1980)	agoraphobic outpatients with panic attacks	45–60	imipramine and placebo	150	12	both drugs superior to placebo; PH consistently more effective than IMI

Nies & Robinson (1981)	outpatients with primary depressive disorder	60	amitriptyline	150	6	both drugs of comparable overall effectiveness; PH superior on atypical features while AMI superior on endogenous features
Rowan et al. (1982)	outpatients with depression or mixed anxiety depression	45–75	amitriptyline and placebo	75–187.5	6	both drugs superior to placebo; PH better on anxiety ratings while AMI better on depression ratings
Liebowitz et al. (1984)	outpatients with atypical depression	60–90	imipramine and placebo	200–300	6	both drugs superior to placebo; no finding of IMI superiority over PH on any measure
Kayser et al. (1985)	outpatients with depression	60	amitriptyline	150	6	patients with high score on hysteroid dysphoria questionnaire showed significantly more improvement with PH than with AMI

effects may show tranylcypromine to be effective in a different group of patients. Two recent studies (McGrath, Quitkin, Harrison, & Stewart, 1984; Nolan, Van de Putten, Dijken, & Kamp, 1985) reported a favorable response to tranylcypromine in patients with major depression who were previously unresponsive to other antidepressant therapy.

The Effect of MAOIs in Patients with Eating Disorders

(a) Bulimia Nervosa

The first apparent description of the use of an MAOI to treat a patient with bulimia nervosa was provided by Rich in 1978. He described a patient who had both bulimia nervosa and a major affective illness, who failed to respond adequately to a tricyclic antidepressant. Treatment with an MAOI led to remission both of the depression and of the eating disturbance. In 1982, Walsh and colleagues described six women of normal weight with bulimia nervosa who also had symptoms of atypical depression, and who showed impressive responses to MAOIs. These encouraging preliminary findings led Walsh and his colleagues to conduct a double-blind, placebo-controlled trial of the MAOI phenelzine in women with bulimia nervosa.

Patients were selected to be of normal weight, to have had bulimia nervosa for at least 1 year, and to be bingeing at least three times per week at time of entry into the study. The study was designed to last 10 weeks. During the first two weeks, all patients were given placebo in single-blind fashion. This phase was designed to eliminate patients who responded to placebo alone, as well as to verify compliance with the tyramine-free diet and with the administrative requirements of the study. Patients who failed to respond to two weeks of single-blind placebo treatment were then randomized either to continue placebo or to receive phenelzine, and were treated for an additional 8 weeks in double-blind fashion.

Results from the first 30 patients who completed the study have been reported (Walsh, Stewart, Roose, Gladis, & Glassman, 1985c) and demonstrate a significant difference between phenelzine and placebo. Whereas patients in both drug- and placebo-treated groups were bingeing approximately 10 times per week at randomization, at the conclusion of the study, patients treated with phenelzine were bingeing, on average, 3.4 times per week vs. 9.1 times per week in the placebo-treated group (p <.01). Six of the 14 phenelzine-treated patients had stopped bingeing entirely compared to none of the placebo-treated patients (p <.01). The score of the phenelzine group on the Eating Attitudes Test was significantly lower than that of the placebo group (23.0 ± 10.6 vs. 44.6 ± 13.2, p <.001). These data suggest that for normal weight women with bulimia nervosa, treatment with the MAOI phenelzine is more effective than placebo, at least over a short-term trial.

Kennedy, Piran, and Garfinkel (1985) recently reported a preliminary trial of isocarboxazid in patients with both restrictive anorexia nervosa and bulimia nervosa. This produced an overall reduction in the frequency of bingeing from 10.2 to 2.4 times per week. In the nonbingeing anorexic group, isocarboxazid showed a trend toward reducing the level of meal restriction, but in neither group was its use associated with any significant alteration in weight. Both groups showed reductions in scales measuring anxiety and depression, adding further fuel to the speculation that antianxiety and antidepressant effects may be contributing to the effect of antidepressants in eating-disorder patients.

This is being tested in a subsequent double-blind placebo-controlled crossover study. So far, of 22 bulimic women entering the 13-week study (six weeks on isocarboxazid and six weeks on placebo with one week for crossover) 13 have completed both phases. During active drug, binges were reduced from an average of 4.6 to 1.5 per week, and vomiting from 5.7 to 2.1 per week while weight remained more or less constant (60.2 kg to 60.4 kg).

During placebo there was also a reduction in binges from 9.4 to 3.4 per week and in vomiting from 8.4 to 5.2 per week. Again, weight remained relatively unchanged (59.5 kg to 60.5 kg).

Levels of monoamine oxidase were measured at the initial visit and at the end of each phase. From this the percentage of enzyme inhibition after six weeks on isocarboxazid was calculated. This provided a measure of drug compliance, and will allow a comparison of therapeutic response with enzyme inhibition at a later stage. Data were available on 12 of the 13 patients. Of these 12, nine had an inhibition value greater than 90%, two were greater than 70%, and one was 37%.

Although the improvement during drug versus placebo is significant, there is a time effect in favor of improvement during the second phase of the study (regardless of whether the individual was on drug or placebo). The higher baseline values for bingeing and vomiting at the onset of placebo are the result of the fact that more patients who completed both phases of the study began on placebo. In fact, seven of the 11 patients who originally started on the drug failed to complete both parts of the study. This may reflect the influence of the other nonspecific therapeutic factors which allowed more patients to continue with six weeks' active drug treatment after forming a "treatment alliance." It may also have been related to the higher incidence of certain additional personality disorder diagnoses in the dropout group. Seven of the dropout group had DSM-III diagnoses of borderline personality disorder compared to only four in the group who completed the study. In addition, the presence of a major depression, or a significant reduction in measures of depression or anxiety was not related to improvement in bulimic symptoms. Hence, preliminary findings suggest that personality disturbances may be particularly important in predicting poor compliance.

(b) Anorexia Nervosa

We also looked separately at the response of five female patients with anorexia nervosa (restrictive subtype) to isocarboxazid under similar double-blind conditions. This was prompted by Davidson's earlier finding (Davidson & Turnbull, 1982) that depressed patients gained or lost weight during successful treatment with isocarboxazid depending on their initial appetite and weight disturbance.

Although only five subjects completed all measures throughout both phases of the study, what stands out most is the overall lack of consistent response during either drug or placebo phase. Only depression and anxiety ratings showed a trend toward improvement in the drug phase. Neither weight gain, evidence of improvement in meal completion, nor repeat measures on the EAT-26 questionnaire showed even a trend toward improvement on the drug. These findings closely resemble the recent negative findings reported by Biederman and colleagues (1985a) who used amitriptyline in the treatment of anorexia nervosa, although two other recent reports (Halmi, Eckert, LaDu, & Cohen, 1986; Hudson, Pope, Jonas, & Yurgelun-Todd, 1985b) offered more modest support for antidepressants as adjunctive treatments. However, the examination of enzyme inhibition data on the five anorexic patients raised concern either about drug absorption, metabolism, or overall compliance. Compared to the mean inhibition of 87% in our bulimic patients, the restricters had an average level of only 48% with a range of 14%–97%.

Side Effects

The major factor that has limited the use of MAOIs, particularly in the United States, has been the danger of hypertensive reactions. When MAOIs were first introduced 30 years ago, the danger of interactions with dietary substances was unknown. A number of serious hypertensive reactions were reported in which patients experienced the sudden onset of excruciating headache associated with high blood pressure, which on rare occasions led to intracranial hemorrhage and death. It was eventually learned that these reactions were caused by the consumption of foods containing vasoactive amines, particularly tyramine, or of medications containing sympathomimetics. As already noted, when care is taken to inform patients of the necessity of dietary adherence, the frequency of hypertensive reactions in the treatment of depressed patients with MAOIs is low (Pare, 1985). However, there is obvious reason for increased concern about the use of MAOIs to treat patients with eating disorders who, by definition, have difficulty controlling their food intake. Thus, the investigators who have described the use of MAOIs in patients with eating disorders have emphasized the necessity of assessing the patients' ability to adhere to a strict tyramine-free diet. Perhaps because of this increased level of vigilance, hypertensive reactions have not proved to be a major problem in the use of MAOIs in the treatment of patients with eating disorders.

Although the MAOIs are probably best recognized for the risk of hypertensive reaction, they are also capable of producing a variety of other less dangerous, but nonetheless problematic side effects. These include reduction in blood pressure leading to postural hypotension and fainting, sleep disturbance, edema, sexual dysfunction, and a variety of minor neurological disturbances including myclonic jerks, paresthesias, and urinary hesitancy. Although these symptoms disappear on discontinuation of the drug, they can be quite troublesome. In a recent survey of drug side effects in a depression clinic, Rabkin and co-workers (1984) found that the MAOI, phenelzine, produced a significantly greater frequency of side effects than did the tricyclic antidepressant, imipramine. Walsh and colleagues (1984) have also reported a high frequency of side effects in their controlled treatment study of phenelzine in normal weight bulimic patients. For example, 10 of 20 patients randomized to phenelzine were unable to complete a full eight-week course because of side effects. Thus, the potential utility of MAOIs in the treatment of patients with eating disorders may be limited by a tendency for these drugs to produce significant side effects.

Clinical Pharmacology

The original hypothesis was that inhibition of MAO increased the availability of monoamines (particularly norepinephrine [NE] and serotonin [5HT]) at central nerve terminals, thus increasing receptor stimulation and producing an antidepressant action. As with other antidepressant agents, there is a time lag of about two weeks before the clinical effect occurs, whereas platelet MAO inhibition may occur within one or two days (Murphy, 1981). More recently, Murphy and colleagues (1984a) have also shown that orthostatic hypotension may occur at the same time as therapeutic effects. They propose that a subsensitivity in the central noradrenergic system may develop over several weeks to account for the action of MAOIs.

Both the NE and 5HT systems have been extensively studied in animal experiments on feeding behavior. As discussed by Goldbloom (Chapter 7), the 5HT system plays a key role in the control of satiety and possibly in macronutrient selection, whereas the NE system appears to mediate amphetamine-induced anorexia. Klein (1974) proposed a disturbance in the regulation of phenylethylamine (PEA), an amphetaminelike substance occurring in the brain during the dysphoria, carbohydrate craving, and hypersomnia of hysteroid dysphorics. However, Murphy and colleagues (1984b), using selective MAOIs, showed that a 50-fold elevation in PEA following treatment with an experimental MAOI, pargyline, did not produce a clinical response. It is therefore unclear whether response to MAOIs in eating disorder patients results from similar or different mechanisms than those tentatively described in depression.

Can MAOI Therapy Be Monitored?

Clinically effective MAOIs are of the irreversible type. This means that the enzyme inhibition is effective until sufficient new enzyme has been generated; for mitochondrial MAO, this is estimated to be between eight to 12 days. Hence it is important to maintain drug and dietary precautions for up to two weeks after stopping MAOI therapy. Unlike the case of some tricyclic antidepressants, plasma levels of the MAOIs have not been related to clinical effect and are not useful in monitoring treatment. Based on the premise that the drugs are metabolized in the liver by acetyl transferase in a similar manner to hydralazine and sulphadimidine, it was proposed that subjects could be classed as fast or slow acetylators. This would imply that fast acetylators need higher doses. Tyrer and associates (1980) compared 45 mg and 90 mg dosages in 60 patients and found no relationship between acetylator status and clinical response. Similarly, Rose (1982) in a review of the subject found only two of seven studies in which treatment outcome was related to acetylator status. Nies (1983) has, in addition, shown that phenelzine may not be acetylated at all.

In contrast, the measurement of platelet MAO inhibition appears to have more clinical relevance. In their study of anxious depression Robinson and colleagues (1978) divided patients retrospectively into those above and below 80% enzyme inhibition during a controlled trial of phenelzine. High inhibition was related to clinical response.

This work suggests that monitoring the level of MAO inhibition may be useful in assessing the adequacy of MAOI treatment. However, it would be helpful to have additional studies of the relationship between MAO inhibition and clinical response in patients with eating disorders before recommending the routine use of laboratory measures of MAO inhibition. Because the degree of enzyme inhibition, at least with phenelzine, appears simply related to dose (Robinson et al., 1978), it may be reasonable to increase the dose until the patient develops an adequate clinical response or intolerable side effects.

Unanswered Questions

Major unanswered questions exist about the role of MAOIs in the treatment of patients with eating disorders. The study of Walsh et al. (1984) demonstrated a significant drug/placebo difference in the treatment of normal weight women with bulimia nervosa. Although this study is supported by uncontrolled reports (Kennedy et al., 1985; Pope, Hudson, & Jonas, 1983), and by the preliminary data of Kennedy's controlled study, firm conclusions about the efficacy of MAOIs in treating bulimia nervosa must await clear confirmation. In underweight patients with anorexia nervosa, only uncontrolled trials of MAOIs have been reported (Hudson et al., 1985b; Kennedy et al., 1985), and these, as well as the preliminary controlled data of Kennedy et al. cited previously, suggest that MAOIs may not be as useful in underweight patients as they are in patients of normal weight.

Several questions are of interest concerning the use of MAOIs in the treatment of normal weight patients with bulimia nervosa. As discussed in Chapter 2, there is evidence that tricyclic antidepressant medication is also of use in the treatment of normal-weight patients with bulimia nervosa. Several authors have described patients who failed to respond to adequate treatment with tricyclics but who did impressively well on MAOIs (Pope et al., 1983; Rich, 1978). However, as we have noted, limited controlled data are available on MAOIs in the treatment of normal-weight patients with bulimia nervosa, and no controlled data whatsoever are available on a direct comparison between tricyclic antidepressants and MAOIs in this patient population. Thus, although there is evidence that MAOIs are of use in the treatment of some normal-weight patients with bulimia nervosa, it is unknown whether MAOIs are more effective in this population than other antidepressant medications.

Another question about the use of MAOIs in normal-weight patients with bulimia nervosa is whether this form of treatment provides additional benefit for patients who are receiving other forms of therapy. There is compelling evidence that nonpharmacological treatment, including behavior modification and cognitive behavioral strategies, are of use to patients with bulimia nervosa although, at present, it is unknown whether there is an advantage in combining MAOIs with nondrug treatments for such patients.

Although it appears that MAOIs may be helpful for some normal-weight patients with bulimia nervosa, it is clear that they are not helpful for all patients. It would be of substantial assistance if we could identify those patients who are particularly likely, or particularly unlikely, to derive benefit from MAOIs. As we have noted, one of the features of bulimia nervosa that prompted psychiatrists to treat this syndrome with MAOIs was the presence of mood disturbance. Hence, it would seem reasonable to expect that the more depressed bulimic subjects would be more likely to respond to medication. Walsh et al. (1985c) stratified their sample at randomization into depressed and nondepressed groups and found a significant difference between drug and placebo in both groups. Similarly, Kennedy et al. (1985) found no relationship between depression and isocarboxazid response. Thus, it appears that some nondepressed patients with bulimia nervosa derive benefit from treatment with MAOIs. The patients who responded to phenelzine also did not differ from the nonresponders in age, duration of illness, or severity of bulimia nervosa. In short, currently it is not possible to predict with any confidence which patients of normal weight with bulimia nervosa are likely to benefit from MAOIs. It is possible that further assessment of personality disturbance in relation to eating disorders may help predict favorable outcome with various treatments including pharmacotherapies.

It is unclear how long those patients who do respond to MAOIs should remain on the drugs. There are hints that the frequency of relapse is high if the medication is discontinued within six months of its initiation, but, at the moment, there are no clear guidelines as to the appropriate length of time the patients who respond to MAOIs for bulimia nervosa should remain on drug.

A final unanswered question is whether newer MAOIs may be advantageous for patients with eating disorders. The recent division of MAO into A and B subtypes (Johnson, 1968) has been followed by the development of selective MAO-Inhibitors. Although the MAOIs currently available (phenelzine, tranylcypromine, and isocarboxazid) are nonselective, clinical trials of an MAO-A selective inhibitor (clorgyline) and an MAO-B inhibitor (deprenyl) have been reported (Lipper, Murphy, Slater, & Buchsbaum, 1979; Mendis, Pare, Sandler, Glover, & Stern, 1981; Murphy, Cohen, Siever, Roy, & Karoum, et al., 1983). Clorgyline appears to have antidepressant and possible antimanic properties (Potter, Murphy, Wehr, Linnoila, & Goodwin, 1982), but has adverse effects similar to currently available MAOIs, including orthostatic hypotension and "the cheese reaction." Deprenyl, on the other hand, does not appear to interact with tyramine but its antidepressant effect has been less clearly demonstrated. At present we are unaware of the use of these drugs in anorexic or bulimic patients, although careful evaluation of these drugs in bulimics may be of research interest.

REFERENCES

Abraham, S. F., & Beumont, P. J. V. How patients describe bulimia or binge eating. *Psychol. Med.,* 12:625-635, 1982.

Ballenger, J., Sheehan, D., & Jacobsen, G. Antidepressant treatment of severe phobic anxiety. Paper presented at the Annual Meeting, American Psychiatric Association, Toronto, May, 1977.

Biederman, J., Rivinus, T. M., Herzog, D. B., Ferber, R. A., Harper, G. P., Orxulak, P. J., Harmatz, J. S., & Schildkraut, J. J. Platelet MAO activity in anorexia nervosa patients with and without a major depressive disorder. *Am. J. Psychiatry,* 141:1244-1247, 1984.

Biederman, J., Herzog, D. B., Rivinus, T.M., Harper, G. P., Ferber, R. A., Rosenbaum, J. F., Harmatz, J. S., Toudorf, R., Orxulak, P. J., & Schildkraut, J. J. Amitriptyline in the treatment of anorexia nervosa: A double blind placebo controlled study. *J. Clin. Psychopharmacology,* 5:10-16, 1985a.

Biederman, J., Rivinus, T., Kemper, K., Hamilton, D., MacFayden, J., & Harmatz, J. Depressive disorders in relatives of anorexia nervosa patients with and without a current episode of nonbipolar major depression. *Am. J. Psychiatry,* 142:1495-1497, 1985b.

Boyar, R. M., Hellman, L. D., Roffwarg, H. P., Katz, J., Zumoff, B., O'Connor, J., Bradlow, H. L., & Fukushima, D. K. Cortisol secretion and metabolism in anorexia nervosa. *New Eng. J. Med.,* 296:190-193, 1977.

Bruch, H. *Eating Disorders.* New York: Basic Books, 1973.

Calabrese, J., Roy, A., Post, R. M., Kellner, C. H., Chrousos, G. P., & Gold, P. W. Corticotropin releasing factor in depression. Presented at the 138th annual meeting of the American Psychiatric Association, Dallas, 1985.

Cantwell, D. P., Sturzenberger, S., Burroughs, J., Salkin, B., & Green, J. K. Anorexia nervosa. An affective disorder? *Arch. Gen. Psychiatry,* 34:1087–1093, 1977.

Carroll, B. J., Feinberg, M., Greden, J. F., Tarika, J., Albala, A. A., Haskett, R. F., James, N. M., Kronfol, Z., Lohr, N., Steiner, M., de Vine, J. P., & Young, E. A specific laboratory test for the diagnosis of melancholia. Standardization, validation, and clinical utility. *Arch. Gen. Psychiatry,* 38:15–22, 1981.

Coble, P., Foster, F. G., & Kupfer, D. J. Electroencephalographic sleep diagnosis of primary depression. *Arch. Gen. Psychiatry,* 33:1124–1127, 1976.

Davidson, J., Weiss, J., Sullivan, J., Turnbull, C., & Linnoila, M. A placebo controlled evaluation of isocarboxazid in outpatients. In M. B. H. Youdim & E. S. Paykel (Eds.), *Monoamine Oxidase Inhibitors. The State of the Art.* Chichester, England: John Wiley, 1981, pp. 115–124.

Davidson, J., & Turnbull, C. Loss of appetite and weight associated with the monoamine oxidase inhibitor isocarboxazid. *J. Clin. Psychopharmacol.,* 2:263–266, 1982.

Davidson, J., & Turnbull, C. Isocarboxazid—efficacy and tolerance. *J. Affec. Dis.,* 5:183–189, 1983.

Fairburn, C. G., & Cooper, P. J. The clinical features of bulimia nervosa. *Br. J. Psychiat.,* 144:238–246, 1984.

Folstein, M. F., Wakeling, A., & De Souza, V. Analogue scale measurement of the symptoms of patients suffering from anorexia nervosa. In R. Vigersky (Ed.), *Anorexia Nervosa.* New York: Raven Press, pp. 21–26, 1977.

Gershon, E. S., Hamovit, J. R., Schreiber, J. L., et al. Anorexia nervosa and major affective disorders associated in families: A preliminary report. In S. B. Guze, F. J. Earls, & J. E. Barretet (Eds.), *Childhood Psychopathology and Development.* New York: Raven Press, 1983, pp. 279–286.

Gershon, E. S., Schreiber, J. L., Hamovit, J. R., Dibble, E. D., Kaye, W., Nurnberger, J. I., Andersen, A., & Ebert, M. Clinical findings in patients with anorexia nervosa and affective illness in their relatives. *Am. J. Psychiatry,* 141:1419–1422, 1984.

Giller, E., Bialos, D., Riddle, M., & Sholomskas, A. Monoamine oxidase inhibitor—responsive depression. *Psychiatry Research,* 6:41-48, 1982.

Gillin, J. C., Duncan, W., Pettigrew, K. D., Frankel, B. L., & Snyder, F. Successful separation of depressed, normal and insomniac subjects by EEG sleep data. *Arch. Gen. Psychiatry,* 36:85-90, 1979.

Glick, B. S. Double-blind study of tranylcypromine and phenelzine in depression. *Dis. Nerv. Syst.,* 25:617-619, 1964.

Gwirtsman, H. E., Roy-Byrne, P., Yager, J., & Gerner, R. H. Neuroendocrine abnormalities in bulimia. *Am. J. Psychiatry,* 140:559-563, 1983.

Halmi, K. A., Goldberg, S. C., Eckert, E., Casper, R., & Davis, J. M. Pretreatment evaluation of anorexia nervosa. In R. Vigersky (Ed.), *Anorexia Nervosa.* New York: Raven Press, pp. 43-54, 1977.

Halmi, K. A., Eckert, E., LaDu, T. J., & Cohen, J. Anorexia nervosa, treatment efficacy of cyproheptadine and amitriptyline. *Arch. Gen. Psychiatry,* 43:177-181, 1986.

Hamilton, M. Drug resistant depressions: response to ECT. *Pharmakopsychiatric Neuro-Psychopharmacologie,* 7:205-206, 1974.

Herzog, D. B. Are anorexic and bulimic patients depressed? *Am. J. Psychiatry,* 141:1594-1597, 1984.

Himmelhoch, J. M., Fuchs, C. Z., & Symons, B. J. A double-blind study of tranylcypromine treatment of major anergic depression. *J. Nerv. and Ment. Dis.,* 170:628-634, 1982.

Hsu, L. K. G. Outcome of anorexia nervosa. A review of the literature (1954 to 1978). *Arch. Gen. Psychiatry,* 37:1041-1046, 1980.

Hudson, J. I., Pope, H. G., & Jonas, J. M. Bulimia: A form of affective disorder? Presented at the Annual Meeting of the American Psychiatric Association, May, 1983a.

Hudson, J. I., Pope, H. G. Jr., Jonas, J. M., & Yurgelun-Todd, D. Family history study of anorexia nervosa and bulimia. *Br. J. Psychiatry,* 142:133-138, 1983b.

Hudson, J. I., Jonas, J. M., Pope, H. G., & Grochochinski, V. Sleep EEG in bulimia. Presented at the Annual Meeting, American Psychiatric Association, May 1985a.

Hudson, J. I., Pope, H. G., Jonas, J. M., & Yurgelun-Todd, D. Treatment of anorexia nervosa with antidepressants. *J. Clin. Psychopharm.,* 5:17-23, 1985b.

Johnson, C., & Larson, R. Bulimia: An analysis of moods and behavior. *Psychom. Med.,* 44:341–355, 1982.

Johnson, J. P. Some observations upon a new inhibitor of monoamine oxidase in brain tissue. *Biochem. Pharmacol.,* 17:1285–1297, 1968.

Johnstone, E. D., & Marsh, W. Acetylator status and response to phenelzine in depressed patients. *Lancet,* 1:567–570, 1973.

Katz, J. L., Kuperberg, A., Pollack, C. P., Walsh, B. T., Zumoff, B., & Weiner, H. Is there a relationship between eating disorder and affective disorder? New evidence from sleep recordings. *Am. J. Psychiatry,* 141:753–758, 1984.

Kayser, A., Robinson, D. S., Nies, A., & Howard, D. Response to phenelzine among depressed patients with feature of hysteroid dysphoria. *Am. J. Psychiatry,* 142:486–488, 1985.

Kelly, D., Guirguis, W., Frommer, E., Mitchell-Heggs, N., & Sargant, W. Treatment of phobic states with antidepressants. *Br. J. Psychiatry,* 116:387–398, 1970.

Kennedy, S. H., Stokl, S., Garfinkel, P. E., Wilkes, B., Stern-Mighton, D., & Piran, N. Effects of weight change on the dexamethasone suppression test. Presented at Canadian Psychiatric Association, 34th Annual Meeting, Banff, 1984.

Kennedy, S. H., Piran, N., & Garfinkel, P. E. Monoamine oxidase inhibitor therapy for anorexia nervosa and bulimia: A preliminary trial of isocarboxazid. *J. Clin. Psychopharmacol.,* 5:279–285, 1985.

Keys, A., Brozek, J., Henschel, A., Mickelsen, O., & Taylor, H. L. *The Biology of Human Starvation.* Minneapolis: University of Minnesota Press, 1950.

Khanna, J. L., Pratt, S., & Burdizk, E. G. A study of certain effects of tranylcypromine, a new antidepressant. *J. New Drugs,* 3:227–232, 1963.

Klein, D. F., & Davis, J. (Eds.). *Diagnosis and Drug Treatment of Psychiatric Disorders* (1st ed.). Baltimore: Williams & Wilkins, 1968.

Klein, D. F. Pathophysiology of depressive syndromes. *Biol. Psychiatry,* 8:119–120, 1974.

Klein, D. F., Gittelman, E. R., Quitkin, F. M., & Rifkin, A. (Eds.). *Diagnosis and Drug Treatment of Psychiatric Disorders: Adults and Children* (2nd ed.). Baltimore: Williams & Wilkins, 1980.

Levy, A. B., Dixon, K. N., Schmidt, H. A., & Nasrallah, H. A. REM latency in anorexia nervosa, bulimia and healthy controls. *Abstracts of American College of Neuropsychopharmacology,* 1985.

Liebowitz, M. R., & Klein, D. F. Hysteroid dysphoria. *Psychiatr. Clin. North Am.,* 2:555-575, 1979.

Liebowitz, M. R., Quitkin, F. M., Stewart, J. W., McGrath, P. J., Harrison, W., Rabkin, J., Tricamo, E., Markowitz, J. S., & Klein, D. F. Phenelzine versus imipramine in atypical depression. *Arch. Gen. Psychiatry,* 41:669-677, 1984.

Lindy, D. C., Walsh, B. T., Roose, S. P., Gladis, M., & Glassman, A. H. The dexamethasone suppression test in bulimia. *Am. J. Psychiatry,* 142(11):1375-1376, 1985.

Lipper, S., Murphy, D. L., Slater, S., & Buchsbaum, M. S. Comparative behavioural effects of clorgyline and pargyline in man. Preliminary evaluation. *Psychopharmacol.,* 62:123-128, 1979.

McGrath, P. J., Quitkin, F. M., Harrison, W., & Stewart, J. W. Treatment of melancholia with tranylcypromine. *Am. J. Psychiatry,* 141:288-289, 1984.

Medical Research Council. Clinical trial of the treatment of depressive illness. *Br. Med. J.,* 1:881-886, 1965.

Mendis, N., Pare, C. M. B., Sandler, M., Glover, V., & Stern, G. M. Is the failure of (−) deprenyl, a selective monoamine oxidase B inhibitor, to alleviate depression related to freedom from the cheese effect? *Psychopharmacol.,* 73:87-90, 1981.

Mountjoy, C. Q., Roth, M., Garside, R. F., & Leitch, I. M. A clinical trial of phenelzine in anxiety depressive and phobic neurosis. *Br. J. Psychiatry,* 131:486-492, 1977.

Murphy, D. L. Clinical, genetic, hormonal and drug influences on the activity of human platelet monoamine oxidase. In *Monoamine Oxidase and Its Inhibition.* Ciba Foundation Symposium 39. Amsterdam, North Holland: Elsevier Excerpta Medica, 1981.

Murphy, D. L., Cohen, R. M., Siever, L. J., Roy, B., Karoum, F., Wyatt, R. J., Garrick, N. A., & Linnoila, M. Clinical and laboratory studies with selective monoamine oxidase inhibiting drugs. *Modern Problems of Pharmacopsychiatry,* 19:287-303, 1983.

Murphy, D. L., Cohen, R. M., Garrick, N., Siever, L. J., & Campbell, I. C. Utilization of substrate selective monoamine oxidase inhibitors to explore neurotransmitter hypotheses of the affective disorders. In R.

M. Post & J. C. Ballenger (Eds.), *Neurobiology of the Mood Disorders*. Baltimore: Williams & Wilkins, 1984a, pp. 710-720.

Murphy, D. L., Sunderland, T., & Cohen, R. M. Monoamine oxidase-inhibiting antidepressants. *Psychiatr. Clin. North Am.,* 7:549-562, 1984b.

Nies, A. Clinical applications of MAOI's. In G. D. Burrows, T. R. Norman, & B. Davies (Eds.), *Drugs in Psychiatry*(1). Amsterdam: Elsevier, 1983, pp. 229-247.

Nies, A., & Robinson, D. S. Comparison of clinical effects of amitriptyline and phenelzine treatment. In M. B. H. Youdim, & E. S. Paykel (Eds.), *Monoamine oxidase inhibitors—the State of the Art*. Chichester, England: John Wiley, 1981, pp. 141-148.

Nolan, W. A., Van de Putten, J. J., Dijken, W. A., & Kamp, J. S. L-5HTP in depression resistant to reuptake inhibitors. An open comparative study with tranylcypromine. *Br. J. Psychiatry,* 147:16-22, 1985.

Pare, C. M. B. The present status of monoamine oxidase inhibitors. *Br. J. Psychiatry,* 146:576-584, 1985.

Piran, N., Kennedy, S., Garfinkel, P. E., & Owens, M. Affective disturbance in eating disorders. *J. Nerv. Ment. Dis.,* 173:395-400, 1985.

Pohl, R., Berchou, R., & Rainey, J. M. Tricyclic antidepressants and monoamine oxidase inhibitors in the treatment of agoraphobia. *J. Clin. Psychopharmacol.,* 2:399-407, 1982.

Pope, H. G., Hudson, J. I., & Jonas, J. M. Antidepressant treatment of bulimia: Preliminary experience and practical recommendations. *J. Clin. Psychopharmacol.,* 3:274-281, 1983.

Potter, W. Z., Murphy, D. L., Wehr, T. A., Linnoila, M., & Goodwin, F. K. Clorgyline. *Arch. Gen. Psychiatry,* 33:505-510, 1982.

Pyle, R. L., Mitchell, J. E., Eckert, E. D. Bulimia: A report of 34 cases. *J. Clin. Psychiatry,* 42:60-64, 1981.

Rabkin, J., Quitkin, F., Harrison, W., Tricamo, E., & McGrath, P. Adverse reactions to monoamine oxidase inhibitors. Part I: A comparative study. *J. Clin. Psychopharmacol.,* 4:270-278, 1984.

Raskin, A., Schulterbrandt, J. G., Reatig, N., Crook, T. H., & Olde, D. Depression subtypes and response to phenelzine, diazepam, and a placebo. *Arch. Gen. Psychiatry,* 30:66-75, 1974.

Ravaris, C. L., Nies, A., Robinson, D. S., Ives, J. O., Lamborn, K. R., & Korson, L. A multiple-dose controlled study of phenelzine in depressive-anxiety states. *Arch. Gen. Psychiatry,* 33:347-350, 1976.

Ravaris, C. L., Robinson, D. S., Ives, J. O., Nies, A., & Bartlett, D. Phenelzine and amitriptyline in the treatment of depression. *Arch. Gen. Psychiatry,* 37:1075-1081, 1980.

Rich, C. L. Self-induced vomiting. Psychiatric considerations. *JAMA,* 239:2688-2689, 1978.

Rivinus, T. M., Biederman, J., Herzog, D. B., Kemper, K., Harper, G. P., Harmatz, J. S., & Houseworth, S. Anorexia nervosa and affective disorders: A controlled family history study. *Am. J. Psychiatry,* 141:1414-1418, 1984.

Robinson, D. S., Nies, A., Ravaris, C. L., Ives, J. O., & Bartlett, D. Clinical psychopharmacology of phenelzine: MAO activity and clinical response. In M. A. Lipton, A. DiMascao, & K. F. Killen (Eds.), *Psychopharmacology: A Generation of Progress.* New York: Raven Press, 1978, pp. 961-973.

Robinson, D. S., Nies, A., Ravaris, C. L., & Lamborn, K. R. The monoamine oxidase inhibitor, phenelzine, in the treatment of depressive-anxiety states. *Arch. Gen. Psychiatry,* 29:407-413, 1973.

Rose, S. The relationship of acetylation phenotype to treatment with MAOI's: A review. *J. Clin. Psychopharmacol.,* 2:161-164, 1982.

Rowan, P. R., Paykel, E. S., & Parker, R. R. Phenelzine and amitriptyline. Effects on symptoms of neurotic depression. *Br. J. Psychiatry,* 140:475-483, 1982.

Russell, G. Bulimia nervosa: An ominous variant of anorexia nervosa. *Psychol. Med.,* 9:429-448, 1979.

Sachar, E. J., Hellman, L., Roffwarg, H. P., Halpern, F. S., Fukushima, D. K., & Gallagher, T. F. Disrupted 24-hour patterns of cortisol secretion in psychotic depression. *Arch. Gen. Psychiatry,* 28:19-24, 1973.

Sargant, W. Drugs in the treatment of depression. *Br. Med. J.,* 1:225-227, 1961.

Sheehan, D. V., Ballenger, J., & Jacobsen, G. Treatment of endogenous anxiety with phobic, hysterical, and hypochondriacal symptoms. *Arch. Gen. Psychiatry,* 37:51-59, 1980.

Solyom, L., Heseltine, G. F. D., McClure, D. J., Solyom, C., Lewidge, B., & Steinberg, D. Behaviour therapy versus drug therapy in the treatment of phobic neurosis. *Can. Psychiatr. Assoc. J.,* 18:25-31, 1973.

Spitzer, R. L., & Williams, J. B. W. Hysteroid dysphoria: An unsuccessful attempt to demonstrate its syndromal validity. *Am. J. Psychiatry,* 139:1286-1291, 1982.

Stern, S. L., Dixon, K. N., Nemzer, E., Lake, M. D., Sansone, R. A., Smeltzer, D. J., Lantz, S., & Schrier, S. S. Affective disorder in the families of women with normal weight bulimia. *Am. J. Psychiatry,* 141:1224-1227, 1984.

Strober, M. The significance of bulimia in juvenile anorexia nervosa: An exploration of possible etiologic factors. *Internat. J. Eat. Dis.,* 1:28-43, 1982.

Strober, M., Salkin, B., Burroughs, J., & Morell, W. Validity of the bulimic-restrictor distinction in anorexia nervosa: Parental personality characteristics and family psychiatric morbidity. *J. Nerv. Ment. Dis.,* 170:345-351, 1982.

Theander, S. Anorexia nervosa: A psychiatric investigation of 94 female patients. *Acta Psychiatr. Scand. Suppl.,* 214, 1970.

Tyrer, P., Candy, J., & Kelly, D. Phenelzine in phobic anxiety: A controlled trial. *Psychol. Med.,* 3:120-124, 1973.

Tyrer, P., Gardner, M., Lambourn, J., & Whitford, M. Clinical and pharmacokinetic factors affecting response to phenelzine. *Br. J. Psychiatry,* 136:359-365, 1980.

Walsh, B. T. Endocrine disturbances in anorexia nervosa and depression. *Psychosomatic Med.,* 44:85-91, 1982.

Walsh, B. T., Stewart, J. W., Wright, L., Harrison, W., Roose, S. P., & Glassman, A. H. Treatment of bulimia with monoamine oxidase inhibitors. *Am. J. Psychiatry,* 139:1629-1630, 1982.

Walsh, B. T., Stewart, J. W., Roose, S. P., Gladis, M., & Glassman, A. H. Treatment of bulimia with phenelzine. A double blind placebo-controlled study. *Arch. Gen. Psychiatry,* 41:1105-1109, 1984.

Walsh, B. T., Goetz, R. R., Roose, S. P., Fingeroth, S., & Glassman, A. H. EEG-monitored sleep in anorexia nervosa and bulimia. *Biol. Psychiatry,* 20:947-956, 1985a.

Walsh, B. T., Roose, S. P., Glassman, A. H., Gladis, M., & Sadik, C. Bulimia and depression. *Psychosomatic Med.,* 47:123-131, 1985b.

Walsh, B. T., Stewart, J. W., Roose, S. P., Gladis, M., & Glassman, A. H. A double-blind trial of phenelzine in bulimia. *J. Psychiat. Res.,* 19:485-489, 1985c.

Walsh, B. T., Roose, S. P., Katz, J. L., Dyrenfurth, I., Wright, L., Vande Wiele, R., & Glassman, A. H. Hypothalamic-pituitary-adrenal activity in anorexia nervosa and bulimia. Submitted for publication, 1986.

Weiss, S. R., & Ebert, M. H. Psychological and behavioral characteristics of normal-weight bulimics and normal-weight controls. *Psychosomatic Med.,* 45:293–303, 1983.

West, E. D., & Dally, P. J. Effects of iproniazid on depressive syndromes. *Br. Med. J.,* 1:1491–1494, 1959.

Winokur, A., March, V., & Mendels, J. Primary affective disorder in relatives of patients with anorexia nervosa. *Am. J. Psychiatry,* 137:695–698, 1980.

Zisook, S. Isocarboxazid in the treatment of depression. *Am. J. Psychiatry,* 140:792–794, 1983.

Zisook, S., Braff, D. L., & Click, M. A. Monoamine oxidase inhibitors in the treatment of atypical depression. *J. Clin. Psychopharm.,* 5:131–137, 1985.

2

Use of Tricyclic Antidepressants in Anorexia Nervosa and Bulimia Nervosa

David B. Herzog and Andrew W. Brotman

Tricyclic antidepressants (TCAs) are commonly used in the treatment of eating disorders. These agents are intended to increase weight gain, reduce bingeing and purging behaviors, diminish anxiety, improve eating attitudes, and decrease depression.

The literature contains substantial evidence suggesting a link between anorexia nervosa, bulimia nervosa, and affective illness. The following are major sources of evidence that relate eating disorders to affective disorders (Herzog, 1984):

1. Eating-disordered patients frequently have current and previous symptoms of affective illness;
2. Eating-disordered patients have higher than expected current and previous episodes of major depressive disorder;
3. Eating-disordered patients seem to have familial aggregation and genetic predisposition to affective disorder;
4. Eating-disordered patients have neuroendocrine abnormalities similar to those found in affective probands;
5. Some eating-disordered patients respond to antidepressant medication.

Depressive symptoms are commonly present in anorexia nervosa and bulimia and have been documented by psychological measures such as the SCL-90 (Weiss & Ebert, 1983). Five studies have assessed major depressive disorder (MDD) in anorexia nervosa and six in bulimia nervosa. One follow-up study found that almost 50% of patients hospitalized for anorexia nervosa met Feighner's criteria for depression (Cantwell, Sturzenberger, & Burroughs, 1977). A retrospective evaluation of case histories of 84 female anorexic patients found that 56% met Research Diagnostic Criteria (RDC) for major depressive disorder and 35% met RDC for endogenous depression (Hendren, 1983). A study of 13 inpatient anorectics showed that 11 (85%) met Feighner's criteria for depression (Viesselman & Roig, 1985), and another study of 13 inpatient restrictive anorexics found that 43% met DSM-III criteria for lifetime diagnosis of major depressive disorder (Halmi, Eckert, & Falk, 1982). At the Massachusetts General Hospital Eating Disorders Unit (EDU) we studied 27 anorexic patients and found that 56% met RDC criteria for major depressive disorder (Herzog, 1984). A study using the NIMH Diagnostic Interview Schedule found that 60% of the bulimic subjects had a lifetime diagnosis of major depression (Hudson, Pope, Jonas, & Yurgelun-Todd, 1983b). In another study of 82 bulimic inpatients, 80% met Feighner's criteria for depression (Viesselman & Roig, 1985). At one eating-disorders clinic, 11% of 108 bulimic women met DSM-III criteria for concomitant MDD (Hatsukami, Eckert, Mitchell, & Pyle, 1984) whereas in another clinic, which is known more for treatment with medication, 30% of 50 bulimic females met criteria for concomitant MDD (Walsh, Roose, Glassman, Gladis, et al., 1985). At the EDU, which is known more for its multidimensional approach, 24% of 55 bulimic females met RDC criteria for major depressive disorder (Herzog, 1984).

Although several family studies document a higher incidence of affective illness and alcoholism in first- and second-degree relatives of anorexics and bulimics (Gershon, Hamovit, Schreiber, Dibble, et al., 1983; Hudson, Pope, & Laffer, 1983a; Rivinus, Biederman, Herzog, Kemper, et al., 1984; Winokur, March, & Mendels, 1980) than in nondepressed controls, more recent studies have challenged those findings (Stern, Dixon, Nemzer, Lake, et al., 1984; Strober, Morrell, Burroughs, Salicia, et al., 1985). However, an increase of eating disorders has not been noted in family studies of depressed subjects (Strober et al., 1985).

Neuroendocrine measures noted to be abnormal in depression have also been found to be abnormal in anorexia nervosa and bulimia. Low excretion of the metabolite 3-methoxy-4 hydroxy phenylglycol (MHPG) (Biederman, Rivinus, Herzog, Ferber, et al., 1984) and decreased platelet monoamine oxidase activity (Biederman et al., 1984) have been observed in anorexic and depressed patients. Various studies have demonstrated that anorectic and bulimic subjects show nonsuppression of their adrenal response when challenged with dexamethasone (Gwirtsman & Gerner, 1981; Hudson et al., 1983b).

These findings suggest an association between eating disorders and depression and have led to the use of antidepressants for the treatment of anorexia nervosa and bulimia.

Tricyclic antidepressant drugs (TCAs) affect catecholamine and indoleamine metabolism and physiology and may have other effects on brain activity; furthermore they are effective in the treatment of depression. The theory behind the use of TCAs is that if eating disorders and depression share common pathophysiological disturbances, TCAs could prove useful in the treatment of eating disorders either by improving the depressive component of the eating disorder or by improving the symptom complex of the eating disorder.

LITERATURE REVIEW

Anorexia Nervosa—Open Studies

The literature describing the treatment of anorexia nervosa with tricyclic and heterocyclic antidepressants is quite sparse for both open and controlled studies. In the late 1970s Moore and White published case reports on the successful treatment of anorexic patients with amitriptyline and imipramine, respectively. They noted that their patients seemed to have a response to modest doses of these drugs by gaining weight, having a decrease in depressive symptoms, and having a decrease in abnormal attitudes toward food (Moore, 1977; White & Schnaultz, 1977).

These case reports seemed to be substantiated by Needleman and Waber, who collected a series of six patients treated with amitriptyline (Needleman & Waber, 1976; Needleman & Waber, 1977). These were all inpatients who took between 75 and 150 mg of the tricyclic each day for between one and three months. All the patients gained weight as inpatients and seemed to have a diminution of depressive symptoms and abnormal eating attitudes while on the medication. On the basis of this small number of cases, many clinicians began to use modest doses of amitriptyline for their anorexic patients, leading to two controlled studies, which will be reviewed later.

Hudson and colleagues recently published their study of another series of nine patients who met criteria for anorexia nervosa, several of whom also had concomitant purging behaviors. The anorexic patients were treated with a number of antidepressant medications, including the tricyclics, trazodone, and the MAO inhibitors. Several of the patients received more than one trial of medication, so that the average patient in their series received at least two consecutive antidepressant trials. The patients were medicated for a duration of between four weeks to 23 months, and the authors found that four of these patients significantly improved by achieving weight gain and having a decrease in depressive symptomatology (Hudson, Pope, Jonas, Yurgelun-Todd, 1985). Interestingly, all four of these responders were diagnosed to have a concomitant affective disorder. The authors found that the MAO inhibitors and trazodone seemed to be the best-tolerated antidepressants, although the tricyclics could sometimes be helpful.

Virtually all patients in these studies were engaged in other psychotherapeutic treatment modalities, and most had been inpatients during some portion of the medication trial. There is a suggestion that anorexic patients with concurrent affective illness may do better on antidepressant medication than anorexics without such disorders. However, the numbers are small, and no generalizable conclusions can be reached from these case reports.

Anorexia Nervosa—Controlled Studies

These earlier case reports led to the conduct of three controlled studies that utilized tricyclic antidepressants. Halmi and colleagues conducted a three-arm study of cyproheptadine versus amitriptyline and placebo (Halmi et al., 1982), Lacey and Crisp conducted a two-arm study of clomipramine versus placebo (Lacey & Crisp, 1980), and Biederman et al. conducted a two-arm study of amitriptyline versus placebo (Biederman, Herzog, Rivinus, Harper, et al., 1985). (See Table 2-1.)

In Halmi's study, 36 patients completed an eight-week course of either amitriptyline, cyproheptadine, or placebo. The dosage of amitriptyline was between 40 and 160 mg/day. There was a trend for amitriptyline to be better than placebo, but overall, cyproheptadine was superior to both amitriptyline and placebo. These patients were all inpatients, and the amitriptyline-treated patients gained weight and had a decrease in their depression scores which bettered placebo, but were not as good as those treated with the serotonin antagonist cyproheptadine.

Biederman and colleagues continued this work by conducting a five-week double-blind study of amitriptyline versus placebo in 25 anorexic patients at doses of 3 mg/kg. Most of these patients were seen as inpatients, and the results were rather discouraging. These investigators did not find amitriptyline to be helpful for either weight gain or treatment of depression. Interestingly, however, a subgroup of these patients with concomitant major depressive disorder were found to have low levels of urinary 3 methoxy 4 hydroxy phenylglycol. The investigators suggested that treatment with a noradrenergic tricyclic might be superior to amitriptyline in this subgroup of depressed anorexics.

Lacey and Crisp (1980) treated 16 anorexic patients for a duration of 10 weeks using a rather low dose of 50 mg of clomipramine per day. They found that the medication had no substantial effect on weight gain when compared with placebo, but the clomipramine-treated patients seemed to have a subjective increase in hunger.

When taken together, the results of these three studies suggest that the tricyclics utilized in controlled trials did not show superiority over placebo for the treatment of anorexia nervosa. Further studies with noradrenergic agents seem to be indicated on the basis of the available literature.

BULIMIA NERVOSA

Over the last several years, the bulimia syndrome has been researched rather aggressively, with tricyclic antidepressants being a common treatment modality. Pope and colleagues published one of the first reports when they openly treated eight patients with a variety of tricyclic antidepressants (Pope & Hudson, 1982). They found that of the eight patients, six (75%) had at least a 50% decrease in bulimic behavior within three weeks of beginning the tricyclic medication, and maintained the response at a two- to six-month follow-up. In two letters to the editor, Mendels reported that four of six bulimic patients responded to open trials of tricyclics (Mendels, 1983), while Roy-Byrne and colleagues reported that five of seven bulimics treated with heterocyclics had a decrease in depression but most did not have a remission in their bulimia nervosa (Roy-Byrne, Gwirtsman, Edelstein, Yager, et al., 1983).

In a subsequent paper, Pope and associates reported on their experience with 65 bulimic patients using a variety of antidepressant agents including tricyclics, MAO inhibitors, trazodone, and multiple drug combinations (Pope, Hudson, & Jonas, 1983). They report-

Table 2-1
Controlled Trials of Tricyclic and Heterocyclic Medications for Anorexia Nervosa and Bulimia Nervosa

Drug	N = completers	Duration (weeks)	Dose	Results	Comments
Anorexia Nervosa					
Amitriptyline (Biederman et al., 1985)	25	5	3mg/kg	− for AN − for depression	mostly inpatients
Clomipramine (Lacey & Crisp, 1980)	16	10	50 mg	− for weight gain, increased hunger	inpatients
Amitriptyline (Halmi et al., 1986)	36	8	40–160 mg	+	3-arm study of cyproheptadine, amitriptyline, and placebo; all patients—cyproheptadine was better than placebo, and amitriptyline was better for depression and weight gain

Bulimia Nervosa

Imipramine (Pope et al., 1983)	19	6	200 mg	+++	at 2-year follow-up, most patients required multiple drug trials in order to sustain or improve response
Desipramine (Hughes et al., 1984)	19	6	200 mg+	+++	limited follow-up data; blood levels improved response
Amitriptyline (Mitchell & Groat, 1984)	32	8	150 mg	+	AMI group had a 70% reduction in bingeing; placebo group had a 52% reduction
Mianserin (Sabine et al., 1983)	36	8	60 mg	—	both groups substantially improved

Legend
 — no better than placebo
+/— equivocal result, not statistically significant
+ statistical trend better than placebo
++ statistically significant, better than placebo
+++ greater than 80% difference between active drug and placebo

ed that slightly more than 90% of these 65 patients were able to achieve a significant reduction in bulimic behavior after a therapeutic trial of an antidepressant. They found that one-third of their patients were able to achieve a full remission in their bulimic behavior for at least one month. However, these initial responses did not necessarily hold over the long term, because most patients required more than one trial of antidepressant and many relapsed while on medication. Approximately 25% of patients treated with tricyclic antidepressants had no response to a therapeutic trial of these medications. Approximately 20% were able to have a remission in their bulimic symptoms for at least one month, and the remainder (55%) had between a 50–75% diminution of bulimic symptoms. Follow-up data were not available, but the authors report that 35–40% of patients were satisfied with the results that they were achieving with tricyclics and, therefore, the remainder of patients were given subsequent trials of medication, many with MAO inhibitors.

These investigators also reported on their experience with 12 therapeutic trials of the nontricyclic trazodone. One-half of the patients had no response to this medication but the other half had between a 50–75% response rate to it. The authors suggest that their experience may underestimate the effectiveness of trazodone because several of these patients were previously tricyclic-resistant. Damiouji and Ferguson (1984) have reported that trazodone may be quite effective in carbohydrate-craving bulimics. They suggest that the serotonin-enhancing effect of this medication has both an antidepressant and an antibulimic effect on carbohydrate-craving bulimics.

Horne has studied the use of buproprion (Horne, 1984), a unicyclic antidepressant, for the treatment of bulimic patients. He treated 17 bulimics with concomitant major depressive disorder with buproprion, all of whom had been previously treatment-resistant to tricyclic medication. He reported that after one month, 15 of the 17 patients had either a partial or a complete remission of their bulimia nervosa, but by the end of six months, five of those 15 patients had relapsed, one because she could not tolerate the side effects of the medication and four others who had a relapse while on medication and dropped out. The antidepressant effect of buprorion in this group was less robust, with only 35% of the group having at least a 50% reduction in their Hamilton rating score at the end of three months.

In an open study in 1984 we reported the results of our experience with 19 therapeutic trials of tricyclic antidepressants and eight trials of trazodone (Brotman, Herzog, & Woods, 1984). Of those patients who had a trial of tricyclic antidepressant, 57% had initial response of decreasing their bulimic behavior by at least one half or more. However, during the course of the follow-up period the majority of those patients either had a relapse or needed to discontinue medication because of side effects, and only one had a long-term sustained response to the medication. With trazodone, of the eight therapeutic trials completed, five or 62% resulted in a significant antibulimic response. Three of those five responses were sustained over time. The monoamine oxidase inhibitors seem to have a somewhat better outcome than the tricyclics and trazodone in our experience.

The McClean group has also reported that nomifensine, a newly approved antidepressant with stimulantlike qualities, may be effective in bulimics (Pope, Herridae, Hudson, Fontaine, & Yurgelun-Todd, 1985). However, drug fever and hepatotoxicity may be associated with this medication.

These preliminary open studies have led to the conduct of four placebo-controlled, double-blind studies with heterocyclic antidepressants. The drugs that have been used in such studies are imipramine, amitriptyline, desipramine, and mianserin (see Table 2-1).

Controlled Trials

Pope and colleagues conducted a six-week study using 200 mg of imipramine on 22 patients with bulimia (Pope et al., 1983). Three patients dropped out during the course of the study so that they were able to analyze 19 patients at the end of six weeks. Of the nine patients who were on the active drug, eight (89%) had a response to the medication. None of the 10 patients on placebo had a response to placebo and seven of the 10 patients who received imipramine openly after the placebo trial had a response to imipramine. The authors recently reported on two-year follow-up data of these patients who were initially treated with imipramine (Pope & Hudson, 1985). They were able to follow 11 of the patients for two years. These 11 patients required an average of 3.5 successive medication trials in order to maintain an improvement of their condition, suggesting that most either had relapses or were unhappy with their response to medication. Of the 11 patients, seven remained improved on medication at the end of two years, one discontinued medication and relapsed, and three were off medication and still in remission the last time they were seen. The rest of the patients were lost to follow-up, but most of them also had at least two to three medication trials after their initial imipramine trial. Four patients moved or were referred for further treatment elsewhere, and five left treatment, but at their last office visit with the investigators, they were all on medication and most were improved.

Hughes and colleagues reported on a six-week study they carried out with 22 nondepressed bulimics, treating them with variable doses of desipramine (Hughes, Wells, & Cunningham, 1984). They found that at the end of six weeks, nine of the 10 desipramine-treated patients improved by 80%, but none of the 12 placebo patients were improved. When placebo patients were openly treated with desipramine, 10 of 12 were reported to have improved. At the end of a 10-week follow-up period, 14 patients remained on desipramine and maintained a good response, an additional five patients discontinued the medication but continued to have a good response, and three patients had a poor response. In this study the authors found that therapeutic blood levels of medication had a significant impact on improving response rate.

Mitchell and colleagues treated 32 patients in an eight-week study using 150 mg of amitriptyline (Mitchell & Groat, 1984). The patients were stratified into depressed and nondepressed groups, with eight patients having a Hamilton score of greater than 20 receiving amitriptyline, eight patients with a high Hamilton score receiving placebo, eight patients with a low Hamilton score receiving amitriptyline, and eight patients with a low Hamilton score receiving placebo. Additionally, all 32 patients received behavioral therapy during the course of the study. The results showed that all groups had a significant improvement with both the active medication and placebo. In terms of depression, Hamilton scores dropped by 12.5 points with amitriptyline, and 6.1 points with placebo. Therefore, amitriptyline had a significant antidepressant effect on these patients versus placebo. In terms of disordered eating behavior, those patients treated with amitriptyline had a 70% mean reduction in their bingeing frequency, whereas those patients on placebo had a 52% reduction, which was not a significant difference. Individual data were not reported. These data were reported with group means, and blood levels were not correlated with improvement. In addition, no follow-up data were provided.

Of interest was the fact that those patients who were more depressed had a poorer response of their eating disorder, as compared to those patients who were less depressed. In Pope's imipramine study, the depressed patients also seemed to do worse, only three of seven having responded to antidepressant medication by having a marked response of their eating disorder. Although this evidence is clearly preliminary, the presence of major depression may be a poor prognostic sign in terms of a bulimia response to antidepressants, even if depression improves while the patient is on medication.

In the final controlled study, Johnson-Sabine and colleagues (1983) treated patients with the antidepressant mianserin, using 60 mg of the medication for eight weeks. This was essentially a negative study with no differences noted between the mianserin and placebo groups. Both groups seemed to improve somewhat during the course of the study, but the antidepressant did not enhance that improvement. No follow-up data or blood level data were given in this study, and the majority of the patients did not meet criteria for major depression.

CRITIQUE OF STUDIES

The most striking fact in a discussion of the efficacy of tricyclic antidepressants for bulimia is that fewer than 250 patients have been reported on, with less than 150 patients taking part in a placebo-controlled double-blind study. The low "n" is compounded by other problems that may be even more significant. The placebo response rate has been widely variable, spanning 0% to more than 50%. It is very difficult to explain this disparity, except to suggest that more patients need to be treated in more centers so that the spread between placebo and active drug can be further documented. The disparity could be caused by the use of different criteria to define bulimia, but it is unlikely that this could explain such major differences. The use of the DSM-IIIR diagnostic criteria will probably help to reduce any discrepancy of inclusion criteria.

Most of the studies do not report how many patients need to be screened in order to reach their n. The studies reporting better results may have stricter inclusion criteria that will eliminate people who are medically unstable, actively suicidal, or previously treatment resistant. Future studies should specifically report on the number of patients who need to be screened in order to reach n, and the number of dropouts occurring during the study. This would be helpful so that the clinician could be able to predict what his or her success rate might be in the office as compared to the efficacy data of the tricyclics in a strict protocol with rigid inclusion and exclusion criteria.

One of the most difficult problems in assessing the outcome of bulimia is the lack of a verifiable outcome measure aside from self-report. Essentially, every outcome study using outpatients ultimately resorts to self-report. The degree to which patients are distorting their clinical situation in various treatment settings is unknown. The patients who wish to please the researcher may initially report a more positive response.

Perhaps the most crying need in these studies is the need for long-term outcome data. It does seem clear that over the short-term, a significant percentage of patients have a diminution of their bulimic behavior with antidepressants. However, it is equally clear that over time these improvements may not hold, leading to multiple sequential trials of medication. Hopefully, longitudinal studies currently in progress will document the outcome of patients with bulimia nervosa, in addition to long-term follow-up showing the outcome of patients who have been treated with psychotropic medication. Long-term outcome studies of anorexia nervosa have consistently shown that short-term treatment, such as behavioral therapy and psychotropic medication trials, although helpful in the short term, have little effect on the long-term outcome of the illness. Some investigators suggest that rates of relapse and the need for sequential medication trials are not very much different from the treatment of patients with major depression, and it could turn out that patients with bulimia nervosa and depressive symptoms or syndromes could represent a population requiring aggressive, ongoing psychopharmacologic intervention. The issue of the relationship of major depression to bulimia nervosa and anorexia nervosa is still unresolved, and further studies stratifying depressed versus nondepressed eating-disordered patients need to be done.

APPROACH TO THE USE OF TCAs IN EATING-DISORDERED PATIENTS

A. Anorexia Nervosa

Anorexic patients often refuse pharmacotherapy, either because of the syntonicity of the disorder, fear of loss of control, fear that taking medication means that they are crazy, or misinformation concerning the effects and side effects of medication (e.g., obesity). Furthermore, their families may also wish to deny that there is a psychiatric disorder that may respond to psychotropic medication and collude with the patients in their refusal to take medication. In addition, these patients are exquisitely sensitive to side effects and frequently report excessive sedation, insomnia, or dizziness, even at very low doses of medication. Thus, it is extremely important to spend time informing the patient about medication and its uses. These patients want to be well informed and the therapist should ally with their cognitive styles and respect their wishes for information. Psychotropic medication should not be employed as the sole treatment modality for anorexia nervosa, but only as an adjunctive therapy in the context of the psychotherapeutic relationship.

We recommend the use of TCAs as the first choice for pharmacotherapy of the anorexic with concomitant major depressive disorder. Additionally, the anorexic with neurovegetative signs (e.g., insomnia) or recurrent dystonic preoccupations or rituals can benefit from a TCA. The choice of the specific agent involves several factors. Amitriptyline is the best studied TCA in anorexia nervosa and has been beneficial in some patients in short-term trials. However, it frequently produces uncomfortable side effects, particularly excessive sedation and anticholinergic effects. Amitriptyline has also been associated with inducing weight gain and carbohydrate craving. Imipramine is a commonly used effective antidepressant that is also sedating and anticholinergic, but has not been well studied in anorexia nervosa.

We generally initiate treatment with either imipramine or desipramine. We tend to favor desipramine as the drug of choice because it is biologically similar to imipramine and is as effective an antidepressant, but produces fewer sedative and anticholinergic effects than either imipramine or amitriptyline. However, desipramine is much more expensive than either imipramine or amitriptyline and this may be an important practical consideration.

Prior to initiating pharmacotherapy, a careful medical assessment of the anorexic patient is indicated. Anorexic patients may present with substantial medical complications including electrolyte disturbances (i.e., hypokalemia), dehydration, bradycardia, hypotension, anemia or leukopenia, or renal compromise. Routine laboratory tests should include a complete blood count, serum electrolytes, liver function tests, blood urea nitrogen, creatinine, thyroid functions, and an electrocardiogram. All metabolic and physiological abnormalities should be at least partially corrected prior to the administration of tricyclics.

We suggest that the patient be started out at a very low dose (i.e., 10 mg or 25 mg of desipramine or imipramine), depending on the patient's weight, and gradually increased to 3 mg per kilo per day over three to four weeks. The medication can be taken all at bedtime or can be given in divided doses if side effects are prominent. In the outpatient setting, the patient should have vital signs checked at least weekly for the first few weeks, and an electrocardiogram should be taken again once the patient reaches a therapeutic blood level. Plasma drug levels should be drawn every other week during the first month to determine whether the patient has taken the medication and whether the dose is adequate. The therapeutic plasma level for desipramine should be greater than 160 ng/milliliter, and for imipramine the sum of the plasma imipramine and desipramine level should be greater than 180 ng/milliliter. Laboratories vary in their ability to perform levels, and selected patients may respond to lower or higher levels. An adequate trial requires four to six weeks of treatment once adequate plasma levels have been achieved.

How does one judge an adequate response? Parameters include weight gain, increased interest in eating, fewer obsessional thoughts and compulsive rituals, reduction in depressive symptomatology, decrease in anxiety, and willingness to participate in a treatment program. We would recommend treatment with TCAs for a minimum of six months after the anorexic symptoms have improved. The prescription for continued antidepressant depressive treatment even after anorexic symptoms remit is in part the result of findings from studies that depressive disorders frequently appear (Cantwell et al., 1977).

B. Bulimia Nervosa

Bulimic patients are also often resistant to accepting psychotropic medication: They express concerns that they may get hooked on the drug, that drugs are an artificial way of treating a problem, that they may get fat, or that taking medication signifies that they are extremely disturbed. We need to inform these patients that TCAs are not addictive, that TCAs may improve the underlying symptoms but are not intended to produce a high, and that some bulimics may gain weight with or without psychotropic medication when their purging subsides. We have found that excessive weight gain and carbohydrate craving are not common side effects among bulimics treated with TCAs. Side effects can frequently be controlled by either reducing the dose or by switching to another medication. We believe that antidepressants plus psychotherapy are more effective than either pharmacotherapy or psychotherapy provided alone in most conditions. We again emphasize, as we did in the treatment of anorexia nervosa, that we do not recommend psychotropic medication as the sole intervention in bulimia nervosa, except in short-term trials (e.g., for a month or two with close supervision), but that medication should be used in the context of a psychotherapeutic relationship. The treatment of eating disorders usually requires a multimodal approach that should be individualized according to the patient's needs.

Bulimic patients require a thorough psychiatric evaluation, particularly because of the common associations with affective illness, anxiety disorders, suicidality, substance use disorders, and severe character pathology. Furthermore, the patient deserves a thorough medical screening because of the potential for serious medical complications, which include electrolyte abnormalities, dehydration, hypocalcemia, and cardiac arrhythmias. Patients who present with concomitant bulimia and anorexia nervosa are at the greatest risk for medical complications, severe psychiatric disorders, and poor prognosis. Patients who are at medical or psychiatric risk who require a trial with a TCA should generally be hospitalized on an appropriate inpatient unit.

We recommend pharmacotherapy for the bulimic who has concomitant major depressive disorder, substantial depressive or anxiety symptomatology, substantial obsessive-compulsive symptomatology, or who has been resistant to the usual psychotherapeutic interventions. We do not recommend administering TCAs in the outpatient setting to bulimics who are unreliable, acutely suicidal, abusing drugs and unwilling to alter that behavior, psychotic, or who have severe character pathology when there is a poor therapeutic alliance. Furthermore, there are a minority of patients whose bulimia has provided the "glue" to a fragmented ego, and such patients may get considerably worse if their bulimic symptoms remit too quickly.

We usually begin drug treatment for bulimia with desipramine or imipramine taken entirely at bedtime. We use the more sedative agent if the patient has difficulty falling asleep. We start with a low dose of 25 mg and gradually increase to about 3.5 mg per kilo per day of body weight by the third week. Imipramine tends to have fewer sedative and anticholinergic side effects than amitriptyline, and desipramine usually has fewer side effects than imipramine. The best time to take imipramine or desipramine is immediately before bedtime since at that time it is unlikely to be lost through purging. We recommend tricyclic plasma levels in order to determine that the medication is being taken and to ensure that the dose is adequate. Again, as with anorexia nervosa, we recommend a trial for six weeks once an adequate drug level has been achieved. We evaluate a response to medication by noting diminution of bingeing and purging behaviors, and a decrease in depressive, obsessive, and anxiety symptoms.

In those patients who do not respond to an adequate trial of a TCA, we usually try another class of antidepressant such as an MAO inhibitor. For those patients who have had a partial response to the drug, or who relapse while on medication, and whose plasma tricyclic level is adequate, we would first raise the dose of the antidepressant to a higher therapeutic level. If there is no improvement, we would switch to a different agent or add an agent such as lithium.

In our and others' experience, some depressed bulimics will get an excellent response from TCAs only with respect to their depression, whereas others will get an excellent response only with respect to their bulimic symptoms. Most bulimics will have some improvement even though less than a third will be "cured," and even a smaller percentage will have a long-term cure.

We recommend that bulimics who have not responded to nondrug therapies should be given a trial of medication. Because of the potential dangers of the medication and the concomitant psychopathology in bulimic patients, TCAs should be prescribed judiciously.

CONCLUSION

Finally, we want to state our position concerning the controversial role of medication in the treatment of eating disorders. The controversy is not whether medication should be used in anorexia nervosa and bulimia nervosa, but rather what is the place of medication in treating these disorders. In the past few years there has been an increasing number of articles on the use of drugs for eating disorders and most of the bulimia studies have reported promising findings. As a result, some investigators have advocated the use of medication as the primary treatment for these disorders and that other treatments be used only for secondary indications. We do not believe that pharmacotherapy should be prescribed as the *only* treatment, but rather that medication has a *place* in the management of specific symptoms in these often treatment-resistant disorders.

REFERENCES

Biederman, J., Rivinus, T. M., Herzog, D. B., Ferber, R. A., Harper, G. P., Orsulak, P. J., Harmatz, J. S., & Schildkraut, J. J. Platelet MAO activity in anorexia nervosa patients with and without a major depressive disorder. *Am. J. Psychiatry,* 141:1244–1247, 1984.

Biederman, J., Herzog, D. B., Rivinus, T. N., Harper, G. P., Ferber, R. A., Rosenbaum, J. F., Harmatz, J. S., Tondorf, R., Orsulak, P., & Schildkraut, J. J. Amitriptyline in the treatment of anorexia nervosa. *J. Clin. Psychopharmacol.,* 5:10–16, 1985.

Brotman, A. W., Herzog, D. B., & Woods, S. W. Antidepressant treatment of bulimia: The relationship between binging and depressive symptomology. *J. Clin. Psychiatry,* 49:7–9, 1984.

Cantwell, D. P., Sturzenberger, S., & Burroughs, J. Anorexia nervosa: An affective disorder? *Arch. Gen. Psychiatry,* 33:1035–1044, 1977.

Damiouji, N. F., & Ferguson, J. M. Treatment of bulimia with trazodone. Presented at the First International Conference on Eating Disorders. New York, April 1984.

Gershon, E. S., Hamovit, J. R., Schreiber, J. L., Dibble, E. D., Kaye, W., Nurnberger, J. I., Andersen, A., & Ebert, M. Anorexia nervosa and major affective disorders associated in families: A preliminary report. In S. B. Guze, F. J. Earls & J. E. Barrett (Eds.), *Childhood Psychopathology and Development.* New York: Raven Press, 1983.

Gwirtsman, H. E., & Gerner, R. H. Neurochemical abnormalities in anorexia nervosa: Similarities to affective disorders. *Biol. Psychiatry,* 16:991–995, 1981.

Halmi, K. A., Eckert, E., & Falk, J. R. Cyproheptadine for anorexia nervosa. (Letter to editor.) *Lancet,* 1357–1358, 1982.

Halmi, K. A., Eckert, E., LaDu, T. J., & Cohen, J. Anorexia nervosa: Treatment efficacy of cyproheptadine and amitriptyline. *Arch. Gen. Psychiatry,* 43(2):177–181, 1986.

Hatsukami, D., Eckert, E., Mitchell, J., & Pyle, R. Affective disorder and substance abuse in women with bulimia. *Psychol. Med.,* 14:701–704, 1984.

Hendren, R. L. Depression in anorexia nervosa. *J. Am. Acad. Child Psychiatry,* 22:59–62, 1983.

Herzog, D. B. Are anorexic and bulimic patients depressed? *Am. J. Psychiatry,* 141:1594–1597, 1984.

Herzog, D. B., & Copeland, P. M. Eating disorders. *New Eng. J. Med.,* 313:295–303, 1985.

Horne, R. Treatment of bulimia with buproprion. Presented at the First International Conference on Eating Disorders. New York, April, 1984.

Hudson, J. I., Pope, H. G., & Laffer, P. S. Hypothalamic-pituitary-adrenal axis hyperactivity in bulimia. *J. Psychiat. Res.,* 8:111–117, 1983a.

Hudson, J. I., Pope, H. G., Jonas, J. M., & Yurgelun-Todd, D. Phenomenologic relationship of eating disorders to major affective disorder. *J. Psychiat. Res.,* 9:345–354, 1983b.

Hudson, J. I., Pope, H. G., Jonas, J. M., & Yurgelun-Todd, D. Treatment of anorexia nervosa with antidepressants. *J. Clin. Psychopharmacol.,* 5:17–23, 1985.

Hughes, P. C., Wells, C. A., & Cunningham, C. J. A controlled trial using desipramine for bulimia. Presented at the 138th Annual Meeting of the American Psychiatric Association, Los Angeles, May 9, 1984.

Lacey, J. H., & Crisp, A. H. Hunger, food intake and weight: The impact of clomipramine on a receding anorexia nervosa population. *Postgrad. Med. J.,* 56:79–85, 1980.

Mendels, J. Eating disorders and antidepressants (letter). *J. Clin. Psychopharmacol.,* 3:59, 1983.

Mitchell, J. E., & Groat, R. A placebo-controlled double trial of amitriptyline in bulimia. *J. Clin. Psychopharmacol.,* 4:186–193, 1984.

Moore, D. C. Amitriptyline therapy in anorexia nervosa. *Am. J. Psychiatry,* 134:1303–1304, 1977.

Needleman, H. L., & Waber, D. Amitriptyline therapy in patients with anorexia nervosa. *Lancet,* 2:580, 1976.

Needleman, H. L., & Waber, D. The use of amitriptyline in anorexia nervosa. In R. A. Vigersky (Ed.), *Anorexia Nervosa.* New York: Raven Press, 1977, pp. 357–361.

Piran, N., Kennedy, S., Garfinkel, P. E., & Owen, S. M. Affective disturbances in eating disorders. *J. Nerv. Ment. Dis.,* 173:395–400, 1985.

Pope, H. G., & Hudson, J. I. Treatment of bulimia with antidepressants. *Psychopharmacol.,* 78:176–179, 1982.

Pope, H. G., Hudson, J. I., & Jonas, J. M. Antidepressant treatment of bulimia: Preliminary experience and practical recommendations. *J. Clin. Psychopharmacol.,* 3:274–281, 1983.

Pope, H. G., Hudson, J. I., Jonas, J. M., & Yurgelun-Todd, D. Treatment of bulimia with imipramine: A double-blind placebo-controlled study. *Am. J. Psychiatry,* 14:554–558, 1983.

Pope, H. G., Herridae, P. L., Hudson, J. I., Fontaine, R., & Yurgelun-Todd, D. Treatment of nomifensine in bulimia. Presented at the 138th Annual Meeting of the American Psychiatric Association, Dallas, 1985.

Pope, H. G., & Hudson, J. I. Biological treatments of eating disorders. In S. W. Emmett (Ed.), *Theory and Treatment of Anorexia Nervosa and Bulimia.* New York: Brunner/Mazel, 1985, pp. 73–92.

Rivinus, T. M., Biederman, J., Herzog, D. B., Kemper, K., Harper, G. P., Harmatz, J. S., & Houseworth, S. Anorexia nervosa and affective disorders: A controlled family history study. *Am. J. Psychiatry,* 141:1414–1418, 1984.

Roy-Byrne, P., Gwirtsman, H., Edelstein, C. K., Yager, J., & Garner, R. H. Eating disorders and antidepressants (letter). *J. Clin. Psychopharmacol.,* 3:61, 1983.

Sabine, E. J., Yonace, A., Farrinston, A. J., Barratt, K. H., & Wakeling, A. Bulimia nervosa: A placebo controlled double-blind therapeutic trial of mianserin. *Br. J. Clin. Pharmacol.,* 15(2):195s–202s, 1983.

Stern, S. L., Dixon, K. N., Nemzer, E., Lake, M. D., Sansone, R. A., Smeltzer, D. S., Lantz, S., & Schrier, S. S. Affective disorder in the families of women with normal weight bulimia. *Am. J. Psychiatry,* 141:1224–1227, 1984.

Strober, M., Morrell, W., Burroughs, J., Salicia, B., & Jacobs, C. A controlled family study of anorexia nervosa. *J. Psych. Res.,* 19(2–3):239–246, 1985.

Viesselman, J. O., & Roig, M. Depression and suicidality in eating disorders. *J. Clin. Psychiatry,* 46:118–124, 1985.

Walsh, B. T., Roose, S. P., Glassman, A. H., Gladis, M., & Sadik, C. Bulimia and depression. *Psychosomatic Med.,* 47:123–131, 1985.

Weiss, S. R., & Ebert, M. Psychological and behavioral characteristics of normal-weight bulimics and normal-weight controls. *Psychol. Med.,* 49:293–303, 1983.

White, J. H., & Schnaultz, N. L. Successful treatment of anorexia nervosa with imipramine. *Dis. Nerv. Syst.,* 38:567–568, 1977.

Winokur, A., March, V., & Mendels, T. Primary affective disorder in relatives of patients with anorexia nervosa. *Am. J. Psychiatry,* 141:1224–1227, 1980.

3

Uses and Potential Misuses of Antianxiety Agents in the Treatment of Anorexia Nervosa and Bulimia Nervosa

Arnold E. Andersen

The first widely accepted description of anorexia nervosa by Morton (1694) included extensive pharmacological suggestions. Clinical experience during the past three centuries suggests that Morton's initial remedies are not very effective, but that other pharmacological agents may play an important role in treatment. The decades between 1920 and 1960 represented the high point in the psychodynamic understanding of anorexia nervosa. The treatment emphasis during these decades was psychoanalytically oriented psychotherapy with little use of medications. Anorexia nervosa was understood to be primarily a defense against sexual and aggressive impulses that fused with immature concepts of reproduction.

Since 1960, some important changes in the understanding and treatment of the eating disorders have taken place. Unitary concepts of origin have given way to a multifactorial understanding. Bulimic symptoms were first recognized to occur in a subgroup of hospitalized anorectic patients but soon were described in a large group of individuals at normal weight. Anorexia nervosa and bulimia nervosa have come to be seen as part of a spectrum of eating disorders (Andersen, 1983). Treatment has become multidimensional with a logical progression through treatment stages (Andersen, 1985). Effectiveness of treatment is now based on multiple measures of outcome (Hsu, 1980). Morbidity and mortality have decreased considerably.

The 25 years since 1960 also represent the modern era of psychopharmacology, beginning with the development of phenothiazines, tricyclic antidepressants, and specific antianxiety agents. Many of these agents have been employed in the treatment of the eating disorders, initially with anorexia nervosa and more recently for bulimia nervosa. The uses of psychopharmacological treatments for anorexia nervosa and bulimia may be conceptualized as springing from several different conceptual categories:

1. *Psychoactive drug treatments as nonspecific methods to increase compliance, decrease fear, and reduce resistance to weight gain:* chlorpromazine (CPZ), and more recently tetrahydrocannabinol (THC). The use of these agents has decreased as more sophisticated and specific psychotherapeutic behavioral and pharmacological methods have been developed.

2. *Drug treatments to increase appetite and weight:* CPZ, THC, and cyproheptadine (CYP). Therapeutic trials of some of these medications were done at times on an empirical basis and at times as a result of the belief that anorexia nervosa is associated with some decrease in appetite. It is unfortunate that the term *anorexia nervosa* means the "loss of appetite." This word *anorexia* has created much confusion in the English language. The German term for anorexia nervosa says in one long word "leanness passion of puberty" and captures, respectively, along with the British term *weight phobia,* the pursuit-of-thinness theme and the fear-of-fatness theme that dually characterize the disorder.

3. *Drug treatments that grow out of beliefs about the origin and nature of the eating disorders:*

   a. Beliefs that bulimia is a kind of *convulsive disorder* have led to the employment of anticonvulsant medications such as di-

phenylhydantoin (DPH). In this case, the consequences of the bulimic disorder, some nonspecific abnormal EEG activity, have been confused with causes of the disorder.
   b. Beliefs that anorexia nervosa or bulimia nervosa are a form of *affective disorder* have led to treatment trials with antidepressants, both tricyclics and monoamine oxidase inhibitors. This has been an active and fruitful line of research. See Chapters 1 and 2 for details.
   c. Beliefs that anorexia nervosa and bulimia nervosa may represent *excesses or deficiencies* of various neurotransmitters or other biochemicals may be the origin of treatment trials employing various psychoactive agents. For example, anorexia nervosa has been conceptualized as a disorder resulting from an excess of a theorized but unproven amphetaminelike substance, making lithium a logical agent for a treatment trial.

4. *Drug treatments to improve parts of the syndromic manifestations of the eating disorders:* Phenothiazines for psychotic symptoms, antidepressants for depressed mood. This use of medications is individualized and represents the employment of these agents much as they would be used in patients without the associated eating disorder.

5. *Empirical treatment trials* vary from "fishing expeditions" to thoughtful but essentially heuristic efforts to change the course of illness. The finding that tricyclic antidepressants may have a specific antibinge potential independent of their effect on mood represents such an empirical finding.

In summary, psychopharmacological agents have been used in the treatment of eating disorders in a variety of ways, the most common being their employment to change patient resistance or to treat either a symptom of the illness or a theorized cause. Crisp (1984) has recently summarized the role of psychopharmacological agents in anorexia nervosa. The use of antianxiety agents in the treatment of eating disorders has not been extensively described in the literature. Our use of these "minor tranquilizers" at the Johns Hopkins Hospital on both inpatient and outpatient services has grown in a gradual way over the past 10 years based on experience with many hundreds of patients. The employment of these antianxiety agents has been primarily adjunctive and empirical, and as part of an integrated team approach to treatment. Despite these qualifying adjectives, antianxiety agents may play an important role in the treatment of eating disorders and their associated syndromes in both the hospitalized and the ambulatory patient.

ANXIETY AND THE GENESIS AND MAINTENANCE OF THE EATING DISORDERS

Anxiety plays a major role in the genesis and maintenance of the eating disorders. Depression and anxiety are the two major dysphoric moods present in anorexia nervosa and bulimia nervosa but most of the recent literature has focused on the depressed mood. Numerous studies have been conducted investigating the nature of the depressive state in the eating disorders and ways to treat the depression. Somewhat less attention has been given to anxiety, perhaps because of the powerful potential for treatment offered by the antidepressant agents. But anxiety is an integral part of the symptomatology of eating disorders and antianxiety agents logically could play a role in their treatment in a variety of ways.

Worries about obesity, anxiety about not meeting sociocultural norms for thinness, and fears of criticism about weight by peers or family are often the triggers for initial dieting efforts. Behind these surface anxieties are other, more fundamental fears about developmental issues, such as changes in body size and shape, and role changes that occur during puberty and later adolescence. Bruch (1978) and Crisp (1980) and others have conceptualized anorexia nervosa as essentially a "phobic avoidance stance" with different terms being used for this stance. Russell (1975) has developed the concept that the psychopathological motif of fear of fatness is an essential diagnostic criterion for anorexia nervosa. Wilson, Hogan, and Mintz (1983) have explored the psychoanalytic understanding of the anxieties surrounding the development of anorexia nervosa.

Anxiety symptoms likewise perpetuate and maintain the anorectic state. Perceptual distortion heightens the anxiety by magnifying the size of the body and the effect of even small amounts of food on weight. Relief of anxiety by, for example, reducing food intake or fasting, is a major reinforcement for maintaining the behaviors of anorexia nervosa. An important goal of treatment is to reverse this association between anxiety relief and food restriction, and to substitute instead the pairing of a normal event, eating, with a relaxed state, replacing the fears of weight gain with the experience of maintaining weight in a normal range. An abstinence model for treatment is not possible as it is for alcohol dependence, so a patient must learn to eat normally without severe anxiety for treatment to be successful. Anorexia nervosa cannot exist without an anxiety state, even though the patient, especially the pure food restrictor, may find it hard to identify any emotions at all.

The therapist for an anorexic patient needs to deal with both state and trait anxiety. In addition to the anxiety integral to the symptomatology of anorexia nervosa, there is usually trait anxiety as a part of the vulnerable personality. Perfectionistic, self-critical individuals with low self-esteem face each new hurdle of life with fears of failing to achieve their impossible expectations. When trait and state anxiety concur, the personal distress experienced by a patient may be enormous.

Relief of anxiety also plays a major role in the onset and perpetuation of bulimia. Initial bingeing usually results from dieting behavior causing food restriction, hunger, and weight loss. The resulting urge to eat provokes a desire to eat, fear of loss of control, and fear of weight gain. Initial attempts to avoid eating are followed by methods to compensate for the resultant binge eating. After binge eating is established as a behavioral pattern, however, the triggers for binge episodes become generalized from hunger to almost any dysphoric state, anxiety being one of the most frequent ones. Anxiety from the persistent hunger of dieting behavior, anxiety as a trigger to binge-eating, and anxiety from actual loss of control of eating are all intimately involved in establishing the bulimic pattern. Relief of anxiety perpetuates the bulimic syndrome by giving the patient partial, short-term relief much as a drug fix does. Trait anxiety may be less frequently present in patients with bulimia, but what anxiety is present from temperament is amplified by another personality characteristic, the increased, sometimes exquisite, sensitivity to any dysphoric state, and the desire to impulsively do almost anything to obtain relief. Patients with a mixture of anorexic and bulimic behaviors appear to suffer the most psychological distress (Mickalide & Andersen, 1985).

GUIDELINES FOR PRACTICE REGARDING THE USE OF ANTIANXIETY AGENTS

Guidelines for practice combine both the suggestions specific for the eating disorders and those appropriate for any situation in which these medications are used. The guidelines are discussed according to treatment context and type of eating disorder.

Anorexia Nervosa—Inpatient Setting

Refeeding starved anorexic patients poses a challenge to treatment teams. We employ a nursing-supervised supportive approach to weight gain in which food is presented as medication. Patients are expected to use their time in the early stages of treatment to understand themselves rather than to control food and weight. Other programs emphasize a more behavioral approach, with specific contingencies for weight gain or loss. Before we began to employ antianxiety agents in the early refeeding stage, we had an interesting experience using a different approach with a chronically starved patient. We gave to this patient a trial of stimulant medication to decrease the tremendous hunger she experienced which was making her very anxious and fearful of starting to eat. The stimulant medication did indeed decrease her appetite moderately and allowed her to eat more and to gain weight. The decrease in the strong urge to eat had made her less anxious about losing control. This experience of increased patient comfort during refeeding by decreasing the strength of the hunger drive led to some practical open trials with antianxiety agents to decrease not the hunger itself, but the anxiety response to the hunger.

Our practice now is to begin treatment with a week of observation during which the program of nursing supervised nutritional rehabilitation is started and much supportive psychotherapy is offered. If after this first week the patient appears very anxious at meals, she is offered a trial of antianxiety medication. We explain the purpose of the medication, using the anxiety-performance curve to illustrate the rationale for anxiety reduction. Patients who find it difficult to identify emotions but clearly look and act anxious often resist suggestions for the use of minor tranquilizers. They are told that the medication will not increase appetite and will not take away their willpower. It will make them less anxious about doing what the healthy part of them wants to do—to eat with less distress and in a more normal manner. We believe that many of the abnormal eating behaviors grow out of the fears of gaining weight and becoming fat.

We begin with 0.5 mg of Lorazepam one hour before meals, two or three times a day. Other short-term agents such as Oxazepam could be employed. Nonhepatically metabolized agents may be best used in chronically starved patients who show abnormal liver functions. If excess drowsiness results, the frequency or the amount of medication may be reduced, for example, to 0.25 mg before meals, or used only once or twice daily. About 50% of our patients accept the use of antianxiety agents, and the average length of use is two-and-one-half weeks. Drowsiness, ataxia, or other side effects are monitored. Patients report that they were able to eat with less distress; they felt less anxious before meals and less guilty afterwards. As the refeeding progresses, we encourage the substitution of other nonpharmacological methods, such as relaxation states, thought stopping, and cognitive therapy techniques. For some patients these medications have considerably lessened the psychological distress from eating.

The other time when antianxiety agents are used with hospitalized anorexic patients is during the maintenance phase when, for the first time, they are exposed to situations that in the past regularly produced disabling anxiety and anorexic symptoms.

Example

Rosa is an 18-year-old young woman who came from a first-generation Italian family, in which birthdays and holidays were associated with eating large amounts of food. Anyone who was not eating heartily tended to be criticized. Before her second visit home for a birthday party, Rosa was given 0.5 mg of lorazepam (Ativan). In addition, she did role-playing on how to handle the situation. These issues were also addressed in family therapy. The antianxiety agent was added because during her first visit home, she had become very anxious, did not eat, had to leave the party, and felt defeated and hopeless about carrying the improvements she had made in hospital into a real-life home environment. The second visit went much more smoothly.

Anorexia Nervosa—Ambulatory Care

Minor tranquilizers are used much less frequently for the weight-gain phase of outpatient treatment. Usually they are used to decrease anticipatory anxiety about expected events that lead to food restriction, or to reduce anxiety in ongoing situations, or to treat associated anxiety disorders that appear to occur more frequently in patients with anorexia nervosa, such as panic disorder. As with the inpatient, the rationale for use is explained, and cautions about side effects are explained.

Example

Christmas at George's home is associated with a large buffet. He began worrying about attending the festivities weeks in advance, with some loss of sleep and anticipatory dieting to "save up" calories for the event. Treatment included thought-stopping, thought-substitution, role-playing, relaxation methods, and antianxiety agents when anxiety became severe. On Christmas Eve, and on Christmas morning, he took 0.5 mg of Lorazepam and was able to enjoy the holiday, eating somewhat reduced amounts of food, but without great distress or the complete fasting he had previously practiced.

Example

Phyllis is a 27-year-old artist who has recovered from anorexia nervosa, but who becomes very anxious about eating in public (fearing she will vomit) or about flying. When she decided to visit her family in California for the first time in several years, she was given a small prescription for antianxiety medication, and practiced taking it twice before leaving, once before eating in a restaurant, and once at home during the evening. She did not experience her usual panic at flying, but noticed some drowsiness after leaving the plane. She planned to fly again whenever necessary. She also noticed that her fear of vomiting in public decreased. She carried one or two tablets in her purse, and rarely had to use them, except once when she experienced a panic attack at her health spa.

Bulimia Nervosa—The Hospitalized Patient

Antianxiety agents are seldom used in the treatment of bulimic patients at normal weight, but are used, as stated previously, with those suffering lowered weight and meeting criteria for anorexia nervosa with bulimic complications. More often, antianxiety agents are tapered, usually in patients who have used them to excess prior to hospitalization. When bulimic patients with alcohol dependence are admitted, the minor tranquilizers are generally used during the alcohol withdrawal stage to prevent delirium tremens as most general hospitals do.

Bulimia Nervosa—The Outpatient Setting

Dysphoric mood states frequently initiate binge episodes in ambulatory patients being treated for bulimia nervosa. Antianxiety medication may be useful in helping these individuals to function normally in anxiety-producing settings. They may regain a sense of control, and diminish their anticipatory anxiety about normal social functions. The ultimate goal is to prevent the buildup of excessive anxiety, to recognize it early, to discharge it in healthy ways, and to tolerate reasonable amounts of anxiety without having to obtain immediate, unwise relief. But while these goals are being pursued, anxiety may continue to disorganize behavior and prevent participation in helpful, enjoyable activities.

Example

Jane, a 23-year-old nurse, was asked to be maid of honor at a friend's wedding. She wanted to participate, but had anxieties about the meals associated with the wedding, and with the public scrutiny during the wedding ceremony. Before the dinner given after the rehearsal, and one hour before the wedding ceremony, she took 0.5 mg of Lorazepam and was able to participate with only moderate anxiety. When she observed herself on the videotape taken of the ceremony, she was surprised that she did not look anxious, even though she felt moderately anxious and worried about others noticing it.

Example

Sam is a 29-year-old weather broadcaster. The night before he attends any family function with his inlaws, he becomes very anxious and has difficulty sleeping. He restricts his food intake before these events and binge-eats afterwards. He is working in psychotherapy to decrease his anger and fear of his relatives and to tolerate some psychological distress. He takes 0.5 mg of Lorazepam or 0.25 mg of Triazolam on the night before these occasions. During a phase when he was separated from his wife, he required about two weeks of almost daily antianxiety medications, but does not need any currently.

In each of these patients, the antianxiety medication serves to decrease anticipatory anxiety, to decrease disabling anxiety in social or work situations which triggers binge-eating, and to regain a sense of control. The appropriate concern in each of these patients is that the medications not produce dependence or short-circuit psychotherapy. When used in a judicious manner, neither of these consequences need occur. Table 3-1 summarizes the uses and potential abuses of these agents in patients with eating disorders.

POTENTIAL MISUSES OF MINOR TRANQUILIZERS

Potential misuses may be divided into patient-related and iatrogenic categories. The patients who are most vulnerable to dependence are the nonpsychologically minded chronic anorexic patient and the bulimic patient with severe personality disorder, especially those with impulsivity and a history of drug or alcohol dependence. Chronic anorexic patients may find that they feel better without knowing why and resist efforts to cut back on prescriptions for these agents. As long as the dosage does not increase, there are few side effects, but a resistance to psychotherapeutic efforts may continue. The bulimic patient with a history of drug dependence may experience an increasing desire for medication. The nonpsychiatrically trained physician may prescribe antianxiety agents as a nonspecific method to increase weight gain, neglecting an integrated program for treatment. The misuses of these agents by doctors generally consist of too little or too much medication, expecting these agents to do on their own more than they reasonably can be

Table 3-1

Uses and Potential Abuses of Antianxiety Agents in the Treatment of Eating Disorders

	Uses*		Potential Misuses	
	Anorexia Nervosa	Bulimia Nervosa	Anorexia Nervosa	Bulimia Nervosa
Inpatient	Decrease anxiety before meals during weight gain phase. (Rare uses: pre-ECT, "amytal" interview, etc.)	Taper off chronic antianxiety medications. Use in alcoholic detoxification.	Avoid as sole treatment of chronic anxiety.	Cautious use in patients with impulse disorders, history of drug abuse or alcoholism.
Outpatient	During or in anticipation of anxiety-producing events that inhibit eating. Occasional use in associated agoraphobic states.	During or in anticipation of anxiety-producing events that increase urge to binge or purge. Use to regain sense of control and decrease dysphoria.	Avoid as sole treatment of chronic anxiety.	Cautious use in patients with impulse disorders, history of drug abuse or alcoholism.

*Note contraindications, cautions, and general principles of use.

asked to do. When syndromes associated with the eating disorders, such as panic attacks, do not respond to short-term use of antianxiety agents combined with other behavioral or psychodynamic techniques, then longer-term agents such as the tricyclic antidepressants should be considered.

GENERAL USE OF THE BENZODIAZEPINES AND INTEGRATED PROGRAMS FOR EATING DISORDERS

Cohen (1983) has recently reviewed the benzodiazepines, describing their general features and principles of use. Recent textbooks of psychopharmacology give additional details about the basic pharmacology and principles of treatment with these agents. Patients benefit from a clear explanation about the potential benefits of minor tranquilizers. Significant subgroups of patients either do not want to use any medication or expect the medication to accomplish unrealistic effects. Our impression is that anorexic patients more often fall into the first category, and bulimic patients into the latter. We describe realistically how these agents can help, and also the most common side effects. Cautions about concomitant use of alcohol or other sedating medications are given, and warnings about not driving or operating heavy equipment if drowsiness occurs are also given. Many patients drive, but not many operate construction equipment. Individuals who have minimized or concealed a past history of drug or alcohol dependence may find their dependence syndromes reemerging after otherwise appropriate prescriptions of antianxiety agents are given.

On the whole, these minor tranquilizers are remarkably safe, with relatively few side effects except some sedation. They are generally used for short-term situations, with specific goals, and in doses adequate to decrease anxiety to *tolerable* levels, although not always to fully abolish anxiety. A tolerance of some anxiety is helpful. Some agents thought to be helpful for the treatment of eating disorders such as antidepressants, THC, CYP, and so on may exert part of their effect through a nonspecific sedation, and therefore act like antianxiety agents.

The most important guideline is: use these medications as part of an integrated program of treatment. Usually we aim to avoid antianxiety agents on a long-term basis, but use them for short, concentrated periods of time when overwhelming life-circumstances occur, or for occasional use in predictable anxiety-producing situations that occur over an indefinite time. High dose, long-term use, with no psychotherapeutic or behavioral treatment, and with abrupt withdrawal constitutes a quartet of contraindications.

SUMMARY

Anxiety plays a major role in the origin and maintenance of eating disorders. The anxiety is of several types including chronic free-floating anxiety, panic anxiety, intermittent, situational-induced anxiety, anticipatory anxiety, and existential anxiety. The sources of these anxieties are multiple, and include personality features, socioculturally induced anxieties about body size and shape, anxiety in the context of stages of development, anxiety from associated syndromes, and anxiety from the experience of normal impulses and drives. Antianxiety agents may play a logical role in the treatment of both anorexia nervosa and bulimia nervosa, when used in an appropriate manner by being integrated into a comprehensive program, and observing the guidelines for uses specific for the eating disorders and the uses of the benzodiazepines in general.

REFERENCES

Andersen, A. E. Anorexia nervosa and bulimia: A spectrum of eating disorders. *J. Adolesc. Health Care*, 4:15–21, 1983.

Andersen, A. E. *Practical Comprehensive Treatment of Anorexia Nervosa and Bulimia.* Baltimore: Johns Hopkins University Press, 1985.

Bruch, H. *The Golden Cage.* Cambridge, MA: Harvard University Press, 1978.

Cohen, S. The benzodiazepines. *Psychiatric Annals,* 13:65–70, 1983.

Crisp, A. H. *Anorexia Nervosa: Let Me Be.* New York: Grune & Stratton, 1980.

Crisp, A. H. Treatment of anorexia nervosa: What can be the role of psychopharmacological agents? In K. M. Pirke & D. Ploog (Eds.), *The Psychobiology of Anorexia Nervosa.* Berlin: Springer-Verlag, 1984.

Hsu, L. K. G. Outcome of anorexia nervosa. *Arch. Gen. Psychiatry,* 37:1041–1046, 1980.

Mickalide, A. D., & Andersen, A. E. Subgroups of anorexia nervosa and bulimia: Validity and utility. *J. Psychiat. Res.,* 19(2/3):121–128, 1985.

Morton, R. *Phthisiologia: Or a Treatise of Consumptions Wherein the Difference, Nature, Causes, Signs and Cure of All Sorts of Consumptions are Explained.* Walford, London: Sam, Smith and Benj., pp. 1694.

Russell, G. F. M. Anorexia nervosa. In *Textbook of Medicine.* Philadelphia: W. B. Saunders, 1975.

Wilson, C. P., Hogan, C. C., & Mintz, I. L. *Fear of Being Fat.* New York: Jason Aronson, 1983.

4

The Use of Neuroleptics in the Treatment of Anorexia Nervosa Patients

Walter Vandereycken

Neuroleptics, or major tranquilizers, are antipsychotic agents comprising, in chemical terms, drugs such as chlorpromazine, thioridazine, fluphenazine, and other derivatives of phenothiazine, as well as derivatives of thioxanthene (e.g., thiothixene), butyrophenones (e.g., haloperidol), and other classes of which some components are mainly used in Europe (e.g., sulpiride). Neuroleptics are thought to act by blocking dopamine receptors in the mesolimbic system of the brain. In addition to this main action, several antipsychotics also reduce, to a varying degree, noradrenergic and serotonergic transmission. They are especially useful in treating hallucinations, delusions, agitation, and disorganized behavior, whether these symptoms result from a schizophrenic disorder, a manic or depressive disorder, or an identifiable organic disease.

The use of neuroleptics in the treatment of anorexia nervosa has been advocated, in the first place, on the basis of simple clinical trials (as is discussed later in this chapter), but also by virtue of various theoretical arguments. Barry and Klawans (1976) hypothesized that increased cerebral dopaminergic activity might account for the major symptoms of anorexia nervosa. Hence, they suggested treatment with selective dopamine-blocking agents. In addition to this biological reasoning, the use of neuroleptics in anorexia nervosa patients has been proposed on nosological grounds. Although some decades ago anorexia nervosa was regarded as a forme fruste of schizophrenia, later on the two conditions were considered as quite distinct from each other (Bruch, 1973). This does not exclude, however, that some anorexic patients may develop schizophrenia or schizophreniform disorders (Hsu, Meltzer, & Crisp, 1981). Other authors have reported that some anorexics display transiently psychotic symptoms at some point in the course of their illness (Grounds, 1982; Hudson, Pope & Jonas, 1984).

These observations have raised the question of whether anorexia nervosa sometimes represents a prepsychotic state. Selvini Palazzoli (1974) described the anorexic's attitude toward her own body as an "intrapsychic paranoia." Indeed, clinicians will often be puzzled by the fact that the body image disturbance in these patients appears to assume delusional proportions (e.g., claiming to feel fat even when very emaciated). Hence, some authors have conceived anorexia nervosa as a subtype of monosymptomatic hypochondriacal psychosis characterized by a single hypochondriacal, delusional system, distinct from the remainder of the personality (Munro, 1980; Munro & Chmara, 1982). For such a single solitary delusion, a neurolepticlike pimozide has been advocated as the drug of choice (Munro, 1978; Trainor, 1980). The concept of monosymptomatic hypochondriasis is sometimes compared with the notion of dysmorphophobia, i.e., a subjective feeling of ugliness, physical defect, or bodily deformation usually regarded as a disturbance in body image (Thomas, 1984). Although dysmorphophobia may be of a delusional nature and, as such, sometimes an indicator of nascent schizophrenia, it is usually thought of as a disorder with an overvalued idea, i.e., an isolated preoccupying belief, neither delusional nor obsessional in nature, which comes to dominate the subject's life (McKenna, 1984).

A similar notion, also applied to anorexia nervosa, is "monoideism" (Kaffman, 1981). In the view of many clinicians, anorexia nervosa resembles an obsessive-compulsive neurosis. Many patients, especially the restricting anorexics, display features of obsessive personalities (e.g., rigidity, perfectionism) including the frequent manifestations of obsessional symptoms other than just the preoccupation with food, weight, or body shape (Solyom, Freeman, & Miles, 1982; Solyom, Freeman, Thomas, & Miles, 1983a,b). It is said, then, that obsessional patients who do not experience their symptoms as ego alien—anorexics are strongly convinced of the rightness and healthiness of their thoughts and feelings—are probably good candidates for a trial with neuroleptics, in particular haloperidol (Ananth, 1985).

Finally, and not surprisingly given the manifold problems in delineating the syndrome from others, some authors (e.g., Masterson, 1977) have speculated that anorexia nervosa constitutes a special form of borderline disorder situated along the ego functions continuum. From a psychobiological viewpoint (Zarr, 1984), it shows a moderate integration deficit (dysregulation of affect and cognitive disorganization) which is especially recognizable through symptoms of bodily preoccupation and somatic hypersensitivity. Low-dose neuroleptic regimens have been used in the treatment of borderline patients, a subgroup of whom appears to be sensitive to these drugs that are quite efficient in controlling their thought disorders (Brinkley, Beitman, & Friedel, 1979).

So, there seem to be enough arguments for justifying the use of neuroleptics in anorexia nervosa patients. But speculations and beliefs do not suffice to convince the practitioner who is expected to act on the basis of well-established clinical experience and solid research. Are there, more specifically, hard facts derived from data in favor of the use of these antipsychotic agents in anorexia nervosa? To answer this question, we now briefly summarize the existing literature on this subject.

PHENOTHIAZINES

Psychiatrists in Great Britain quite often prescribe neuroleptics for anorexia nervosa patients (Bhanji, 1979). As early as the late

1950s, shortly after its introduction for the treatment of schizophrenia, chlorpromazine was recommended as a "new treatment" for anorexia nervosa. After an initial case presentation (Dally, Oppenheim, & Sargant, 1958) suggested the possible efficacy of such treatment, Dally and Sargant (1960) reported a comparative study on its use. Twenty hospitalized anorexia nervosa patients were treated with chlorpromazine (dosages from 150 to 1000 mg per day) and, simultaneously, were given 40–80 units of insulin in order to stimulate their appetite. During this trial (23–47 days) patients were placed on bed rest and received a high-calorie diet. The results of this regimen were compared with those of a control group of 24 patients who had been treated without drugs over years prior to this study. The chlorpromazine group showed a greater and more rapid weight gain and hence a shorter duration of hospitalization. At follow-up (from three months to three years after discharge), however, group differences in outcome were no longer apparent. Equal numbers of both groups (about one-third) required readmission to the hospital, whereas an increased frequency of postdischarge bulimia nervosa and a longer period for menstruation to return were observed in the chlorpromazine-treated patients. Although it was impossible to isolate which factor was responsible for the short-term effects, Dally and Sargant (1960) originally felt it was the combination of chlorpromazine and insulin. Later, Dally and Sargant (1966) suggested that the neuroleptic was efficient on its own: the weight gain was attributed to the drug overcoming the patient's resistance to food and panic at the prospect of eating. They still recommended high dosage, beginning with oral doses of 150 mg per day and then increasing to 1–1.5 g daily if the patient could tolerate it.

Convinced by a successful trial in a male anorexic (Crisp & Roberts, 1962), Crisp (1965) recommended the use of chlorpromazine, albeit in much smaller doses (400–600 mg/day) and merely as an adjunct to supportive psychotherapy. Again, in Crisp's regimen, drug treatment was combined with mandatory bed rest (and also with nursing encouragement). It has been suggested that, in fact, this combination of rest and sedation might have facilitated weight gain through decreased caloric expenditure (Kuhn, 1969). Another explanation, now from a learning theory viewpoint, supposes that the treatment program included covert elements of operant conditioning (see, e.g., Halmi, 1980): bed rest deprived the patients of their physical (hyper)activity—a restriction they experienced as a punishment—and weight gain was then the only way to reobtain the mobility they liked so much (the learning principle of escape conditioning or negative reinforcement). Blinder, Freeman, and Stunkard (1970) even made the decreasing dose of chlorpromazine contingent upon weight gain and found it was a powerful reinforcer!

Crisp (1984) became aware of the fact that the chlorpromazine he used in the early 1960s had very little direct effect on appetite or ingestion but had probably rendered the patients more compliant, muting their ambivalence about treatment, and less active, having conferred extrapyramidal immobility upon them. Other drug effects that may have contributed to the weight gain in anorexics treated with chlorpromazine are increased fluid intake (or altered fluid balance) and decreased utilization (reduction of resting metabolism, overall activity, and energy expenditure). Ten years after his first experiments with chlorpromazine, Crisp abandoned that approach and, ever since, he has rarely used any drug treatment (Crisp, 1984).

In the meantime, use of chlorpromazine or other phenothiazines in treating anorexia nervosa patients spread all over the world: from the United Kingdom to Germany (Frahm, 1966), the Netherlands (Lafeber, 1971), France (Volmat, Allers, Vittouris, & Dufay, 1970), India (Ghafoor & Ravindranath, 1969), and the United States (see the following). In the 1970s, however, the British psychiatrists who had advocated the use of chlorpromazine became more prudent. Whereas Crisp almost completely stopped its use as mentioned previously, Dally still continued the prescription but only in 30% of the patients, " . . . mainly in the older and middle-age ranges who were restless and anxious and could not be 'persuaded' to eat by 'unending patience' on the part of the nursing staff" (Dally & Gomez,

1979, p. 114). In Germany, phenothiazines are still widely used especially in combination with bed rest and tube feeding, a regimen known there as the Frahm method (Engel & Meyer, 1982; Frahm, 1973; Niederhoff, Wiesler, & Künzer, 1975). Although the use of antidepressants for treating eating-disordered patients became more popular during the last decade, phenothiazines continue to be recommended by several clinicians in the United States and Canada. According to Halmi (1983), chlorpromazine is particularly effective in the severely obsessive-compulsive anorexic patients. For Sours (1980) it is the drug of choice in older patients, especially middle-aged women who, because of extreme anxiety, resist refeeding. Gross (1982) prefers a combination of perphenazine and amitriptyline (a tricyclic antidepressant), although he warns against the many possible side effects and, therefore, advocates low dosages and limited periods of drug treatment. Finally, Garfinkel and Garner (1982) consider chlorpromazine (not more than 300 mg/day) as useful during the initial refeeding period "for the minority of patients who show marked anxiety to foods and inability to eat after the general supportive measures have been attempted" (p. 144).

But, after all, what is the real usefulness of chlorpromazine and other phenothiazines in the treatment of anorexia nervosa patients? These drugs appear to have certain advantages (Garfinkel & Garner, 1982):

- their anxiety-reducing effect may help the patient to overcome the fear of eating and weight gain;
- their sedating effect may be beneficial in restless and unusually hyperactive patients, especially if they have to tolerate bedrest (and artificial feeding) because of vital risks;
- their side effect of increasing weight is wanted in these patients (though the real mode of action is not fully understood).

Chlorpromazine (as well as other phenothiazines) appears to have many disadvantages (Dally & Gomez, 1979; Garfinkel & Garner, 1982; Gross, 1982):

- it lowers the already low blood pressure (orthostatic hypotension) and reduces the already low body temperature;
- it may aggravate leukopenia and can induce agranulocytosis and hemolytic anemia;
- it reduces the convulsive threshold (i.e., increasing incidence of epileptic seizures) and may provoke bulimialike overeating;
- it may induce hyperprolactinemia and delay the return of normal menstrual function;
- it may lead to parkinsonian dyskinetic reactions;
- it can alter the fluid balance and increase the tendency toward constipation with the possibility of obscuring the development of paralytic type of bowel obstruction (ileus);
- it could cause abnormalities in the results of liver function tests whereas liver dysfunctioning may occur as a result of severe malnutrition;
- it might induce fever and sensitivity to the drug (including rash).

From a clinician's point of view this cost/benefit balance is clearly negative. But why then do so many practitioners continue to recommend this type of drug for anorexia nervosa patients? This is the more surprising in light of the fact that, according to modern standards of drug research, there are no solid data to endorse such a recommendation. In fact, as we stated elsewhere (Vandereycken & Meermann, 1984), we are still puzzled by the following question: Is it in spite or because of its popularity that the proclaimed efficacy of chlorpromazine in anorexia nervosa is still lacking real research evidence?

OTHER NEUROLEPTICS

As mentioned previously, Barry and Klawans (1976) suggested treating anorexia nervosa patients with a selective dopamine-blocking drug like *pimozide,* a derivative of the diphenylbutylpiperidine group. Plantey (1977) briefly reported on the "dramatic" improvement with pimozide in a 17-year-old male anorexic patient; within three weeks he gained 20 pounds and his previously implacable obsession with his body weight disappeared, as did his overactivity. Hoes (1980) described beneficial short-term effects of pimozide (combined with copper sulphate) in eight anorexia nervosa patients. Although it was an open and uncontrolled investigation, Hoes seemed to be convinced that pimozide (even in low daily dosage of 1 mg) could induce symptomatic improvement in anorexics.

Encouraged by these reports, Vandereycken and Pierloot (1982, 1983) wondered if their behavioral management program for anorexia nervosa patients could be improved by combining it with the administration of pimozide. Therefore, they conducted a double-blind, placebo-controlled crossover study. After a baseline period of about one week, the patients started medication periods of three weeks, alternating placebo and pimozide (the sequence being randomly allocated). Nine patients received a single daily dose of 4 mg and the nine others 6 mg; all patients were treated on the same ward with a uniform contingency contracting program. Also, body weight, behavioral, and attitudinal variables were regularly assessed by means of an observation scale filled in by the nurses. Although pimozide appeared to be associated with greater weight gain in the beginning, this effect did not reach statistical significance. Some changes were found on the observation scale in favor of the drug (e.g., better attitude toward treatment), but the differences had little clinical significance. Since they did not find clear-cut evidence for the efficacy of pimozide in anorexia nervosa patients, Vandereycken and Pierloot (1982, 1983) did not recommend the use of this neuroleptic drug.

This negative result has been confirmed in other studies. Larkin et al. (1984) entered 24 inpatient anorexics into a random sequential trial in 12 active-placebo pairs during four weeks. No differences were found on a series of clinical ratings and self-reporting questionnaires. Recently, Weizman, Tyano, Wijsenbeek, & Ben David (1985) reported a comparison between behavior therapy and pimozide treatment in 10 anorexia nervosa patients (randomly assigned in two groups). Both treatment modalities were conducted for a period of 20 weeks during which body weight and serum prolactin levels were monitored weekly. An elevation of serum prolactin (i.e., an indicator of antidopaminergic activity) was found only in the five patients treated with pimozide (3 mg per day). Both groups showed a gradual increase in body weight without any significant difference. The authors conclude that their results do not encourage the use of pimozide in anorexia nervosa: the drug treatment is not superior to behavior therapy and may have side effects similar to other neuroleptics. Weizman et al. (1985) mention, for instance, the induction of marked hyperprolactinemia, which might interfere with luteinizing hormone release. Vandereycken and Pierloot (1982, 1983) noticed considerable dyskinetic reactions in an anorexic patient receiving 6 mg pimozide. Finally, Larkin, Conroy, and Walsh (1984) reported high levels of undesirable side effects of pimozide including incapacitation by drowsiness and dizziness, as well as one epileptic seizure. Such an epileptogenic effect of pimozide is rare, but anorexia nervosa patients may be more prone to drug-induced seizures (Dally & Gomez, 1979). In any case, Larkin (1983) drew attention to this considerable risk in a separate short note describing the case mentioned previously (the patient showed a grand mal epileptic seizure when receiving 4 mg pimozide). In conclusion, pimozide does not appear to be of clinical value in anorexia nervosa.

The same conclusion applies to the use of *sulpiride,* a substituted benzamide drug, which is also a selective dopamine antagonist with an antiemetic effect and a beneficial action on mood and appetite in depressives. Some open trials with sulpiride, especially in France, showed a positive effect on appetite, weight increase, and gastrointestinal functioning in patients (mostly children) with psychogenic loss of appetite and/or malnutrition (Dan & Niang, 1973; Desbuquois, Vialatte, Paupe, & Rossignol, 1969; Marchelli, Vaucheret, &

Gómez de Martin Borado, 1973; Martin, Masson, & Thouvenot, 1970; Piennes, 1977; Rouger, 1979). Because of these characteristics, Vandereycken (1984) decided to investigate sulpiride in anorexia nervosa patients in a way similar to his pimozide study, which we discussed previously: a double-blind, placebo-controlled crossover investigation in 18 female inpatients (13 receiving a daily dose of 300 mg and five patients received 400 mg). No direct effect of sulpiride was established with regard to behavioral and attitudinal characteristics as measured by behavior observation scales and self-report questionnaires (including the Eating Attitudes Test). Regarding daily weight gain, sulpiride was, on the whole, superior to placebo, especially during the first three weeks, but this effect did not reach statistical significance. Though no patient had reported untoward effects of the drug, one of the well-known inconveniences of sulpiride is its particular property of increasing serum prolactin levels, causing amenorrhea-galactorrhea in women.

Finally, Munford (1980) described a single-subject experimental analysis to assess the effects of haloperidol and contingency management on weight gain and hyperactivity in a 17-year-old hospitalized anorexic female. Although the study attempted to observe the separate effects of pharmacotherapy and behavioral therapy, the results did not permit firm conclusions regarding the relative contributions of these variables.

CONCLUSION

We are struck by the fact that so many clinicians continue to use phenothiazines such as chlorpromazine, although there is no research evidence of their usefulness in the treatment of anorexia nervosa. The few methodologically acceptable studies on neuroleptics in these patients concern the use of pimozide and sulpiride, but no significant clinical value of these drugs for the treatment of anorexics has been proved so far. Some practitioners may recommend the use of neuroleptics for the short-term relief of anxiety in anorexia nervosa patients who otherwise feel blocked by a strong fear of eating or weight gain. But such patients, first of all, need psychotherapeutic help, and if additional pharmacotherapy is required for anxiolytic purposes, minor tranquilizers should be the drugs of choice (see Andersen's Chapter 3 in this book). Other clinicians may argue that they have obtained considerable weight gain in emaciated anorexia nervosa patients treated with neuroleptics. But even when their experiences could be confirmed, similar or even better results of short-term weight gain can be achieved by behavior therapy programs or medical regimens including bed rest and skilled nursing without drug therapy (Vandereycken & Meermann, 1984).

So we do not need medication to enhance this effect of weight gain and certainly not when such pharmacotherapy is associated with a substantial risk of inducing undesirable or even dangerous side effects. Moreover, the possible beneficial effect of the neuroleptic treatment is still to be considered in a narrow scope: short-term weight restoration. The test of treatment efficacy in anorexia nervosa patients does not rest in the statistics of weight gain, but in the patient's ability to master eating behavior and to develop a positive self-concept as reflected by long-term maintenance of both physical health and psychological integrity. For this purpose, neuroleptics appear to be of little or no benefit and have, thus far, not enhanced our understanding of the underlying pathogenesis in anorexia nervosa.

REFERENCES

Ananth, J. Pharmacotherapy of obsessive-compulsive disorder. In M. Mavissakalian, S. M. Turner, & L. Michelson (Eds.), *Obsessive-Compulsive Disorder.* New York: Plenum Press, 1985, pp. 167–211.

Barry, V. C., & Klawans, H. L. On the role of dopamine in the pathophysiology of anorexia nervosa. *J. Neur. Transmis.,* 38:107–122, 1976.

Bhanji, S. Anorexia nervosa: Physicians' and psychiatrists' opinion and practice. *J. Psychosom. Res.,* 23:7–11, 1979.

Blinder, B. J., Freeman, D. M. A., & Stunkard, A. J. Behavior therapy of anorexia nervosa: Effectiveness of activity as a reinforcer of weight gain. *Am. J. Psychiatry*, 126:1093–1098, 1970.

Brinkley, J. R., Beitman, B. D., & Friedel, R. O. Low-dose neuroleptic regimens in the treatment of borderline patients. *Arch. Gen. Psychiatry*, 36:319–326, 1979.

Bruch, H. *Eating Disorders. Obesity, Anorexia Nervosa, and the Person Within.* New York: Basic Books, 1973.

Condon, J. T. Long-term neuroleptic therapy in chronic anorexia nervosa complicated by tardive dyskinesia. *Acta Psychiat. Scand.*, 73:203–206, 1986.

Crisp, A. H. Clinical and therapeutic aspects of anorexia nervosa—A study of thirty cases. *J. Psychosom. Res.*, 9:67–78, 1965.

Crisp, A. H. Treatment of anorexia nervosa: What can be the role of psychopharmacological agents? In K. M. Pirke & D. Ploog (Eds.), *The Psychobiology of Anorexia Nervosa*. Berlin-New York: Springer-Verlag, 1984, pp. 148–160.

Crisp, A. H., & Roberts, F. J. A case of anorexia nervosa in a male. *Postgrad. Med. J.*, 38:350–353, 1962.

Dally, P., & Gomez, J. *Anorexia Nervosa*. London: William Heinemann, 1979.

Dally, P. J., Oppenheim, G. B., & Sargant, W. Anorexia nervosa. *Br. Med. J.*, 2:633–634, 1958.

Dally, P. J., & Sargant, W. A new treatment of anorexia nervosa. *Br. Med. J.*, 1:1770–1773, 1960.

Dally, P. J., & Sargant, W. Treatment and outcome of anorexia nervosa. *Br. Med. J.*, 2:793–795, 1966.

Dan, V., & Niang, I. Les effets du sulpiride dans les états de dénutrition en milieu hospitalier. *Méd. Afr. Noire*, 20(12):2–11, 1973.

Desbuquois, G., Vialatte, J., Paupe, J., & Rossignol, C. Effets antiémétiques et eutrophiques du sulpiride chez l'enfant. *Ann. Péd.*, 16:460–464, 1969.

Engel, K., & Meyer, A. E. Theorie und Empirie einer mehrfaktoriellen stationären Anorexietherapie für schwer erkrankte Patienten. *Med. Welt*, 33:1812–1816, 1982.

Frahm, H. Beschreibung und Ergebnisse einer somatisch orienterten Behandlung von Kranken mit Anorexia nervosa. *Med. Welt*, 17:2004–2011, 2068–2074, 1966.

Frahm, H. Anorexia nervosa. In H. Hornbostel (Ed.), *Innere Medizin in Praxis und Klinik. Band 4.* Stuttgart: Georg Thieme, 1973, pp. 13-19.

Garfinkel, P. E., & Garner, D. M. *Anorexia Nervosa: A Multidimensional Perspective.* New York: Brunner/Mazel, 1982.

Ghafoor, P. K. A., & Ravindranath, Treatment of anorexia nervosa with chlorpromazine and modified insulin therapy. *J. Ass. Physicians (India),* 17:369-372, 1969.

Gross, M. An in-hospital therapy program. In M. Gross (Ed.), *Anorexia Nervosa. A Comprehensive Approach.* Lexington, MA: Collamore Press, pp. 91-101, 1982.

Grounds, A. Transient psychoses in anorexia nervosa: A report of 7 cases. *Psychol. Med.,* 12:107-113, 1982.

Gwirtsman, H., Kaye, W., Weintraub, M., & Jimerson, D. C. Pharmacologic treatment of eating disorders. *Psychiat. Clin. North Am.,* 7:863-878, 1984.

Halmi, K. A. Anorexia nervosa. In H. I. Kaplan, A. M. Freedman, & B. J. Sadock (Eds.), *Comprehensive Textbook of Psychiatry, III.* Baltimore: Williams & Wilkins, 1980, pp. 1882-1891.

Halmi, K. A. Anorexia nervosa. In H. Hippius & G. Winokur (Eds.), *Psychopharmacology 1. Part 2: Clinical Psychopharmacology.* Amsterdam: Excerpta Medica, 1983, pp. 313-320.

Hoes, M.J.A.J.M. Copper sulphate and pimozide in anorexia nervosa. *J. Orthomol. Psychiatry,* 9:48-51, 1980.

How, J., & Davidson, R.J.L. Chlorpromazine-induced haemolytic anaemia in anorexia nervosa. *Postgrad. Med. J.,* 53:278-279, 1977.

Hsu, L.K.G., Meltzer, E. S., & Crisp, A. H. Schizophrenia and anorexia nervosa. *J. Nerv. Ment. Dis.,* 169:273-276, 1981.

Hudson, J. I., Pope, H. G., & Jonas, J. M. Psychosis in anorexia nervosa and bulimia. *Br. J. Psychiatry,* 145:420-423, 1984.

Johnson, C., Stuckey, M., & Mitchell, J. Psychopharmacological treatment of anorexia nervosa and bulimia. *J. Nerv. Ment. Dis.,* 171:524-534, 1983.

Johnson, C., Stuckey, M., & Mitchell, J. Psychopharmacology of anorexia nervosa and bulimia. In J. E. Mitchell (Ed.), *Anorexia Nervosa and Bulimia. Diagnosis and Treatment.* Minneapolis: University of Minnesota Press, 1985, pp. 134-151.

Kaffman, M. Monoideism in psychiatry: Theoretical and clinical aspects. *Am. J. Psychother.,* 35:235–243, 1981.

Kuhn, R. Psychopathology, pharmacotherapy and psychotherapy of anorexia nervosa. In A. Pletscher, A. Marino, & P. Pinkerton (Eds.), *Psychotropic Drugs in Internal Medicine.* Amsterdam: Excerpta Medica, 1969, pp. 74–79.

Lafeber, C. *Anorexia Nervosa.* Leiden: Stafleu, 1971.

Larkin, C. Epileptogenic effect of pimozide (letter). *Am. J. Psychiatry,* 140:372–373, 1983.

Larkin, C., Conroy, R., & Walsh, N. A double-blind controlled trial of pimozide in body-image disorder in anorexia nervosa. Paper read at the International Conference on Anorexia Nervosa and Related Disorders, Swansea, England, September 3–7, 1984.

Marchelli, E. A., Vaucheret, G., & Gómez de Martin Borado, H. Tratamiento de la anorexia nerviosa con sulpiride. *Rev. Argent. Psicofarmacol.,* April–June, 14–17, 1973.

Martin, A., Masson, J. M., & Thouvenot, J. L'électrosplanchnographie dans les anorexies mentales et les dépressions. Premiers résultats. *Sem. Hôp. Paris,* 46(29B):54–60, 1970.

Masterson, J. F. Primary anorexia nervosa in the borderline adolescent— An object-relations view. In P. Hartocollis (Ed.), *Borderline Personality Disorders.* New York: International Universities Press, 1977, pp. 475–494.

McKenna, P. J. Disorders with overvalued ideas. *Br. J. Psychiatry,* 145:579–585, 1984.

Meermann, R. Zur Psychopharmakotherapie der Anorexia nervosa. *Prax. Psychother. Psychosom.,* 25:269–278, 1980.

Meermann, R. Zur Psychopharmakotherapie der Magersucht. In R. Meermann (Ed.), *Anorexia Nervosa. Ursachen und Behandlung.* Stuttgart: Ferdinand Enke, 1981, pp. 170–178.

Munford, P. R. Haloperidol and contingency management in a case of anorexia nervosa. *J. Behav. Ther. Exp. Psychiatry,* 11:67–72, 1980.

Munro, A. Monosymptomatic hypochondriacal psychosis. A diagnostic entity which may respond to pimozide. *Can. Psychiat. Ass. J.,* 23:497–500, 1978.

Munro, A. Monosymptomatic hypochondriacal psychosis. *Br. J. Hosp. Med.,* 24:34–38, 1980. Reprinted in S. Crown (Ed.), *Contemporary Psy-*

chiatry. London: Butterworths, 1984, pp. 80–88.

Munro, A., & Chmara, J. Monosymptomatic hypochondriacal psychosis. *Can. J. Psychiatry,* 27:374–376, 1982.

Niederhoff, H., Wiesler, B., & Künzer, W. Somatisch orientierte Behandlung der Anorexia nervosa. *Mschr. Kinderheilk.,* 123:343–344, 1975.

Piennes, M. G. L'intérêt du Dogmatil dans le traitement de l'anorexie mentale de l'enfant. *J. Méd. Chir. Prat.,* 148:201–203, 1977.

Plantey, F. Pimozide in treatment of anorexia nervosa (letter). *Lancet,* 1:1105, 1977.

Rouger, M. E. A propos de l'effet orexigène du sulpiride. *J. Méd. Chir. Prat.,* 150:452–457, 1979.

Selvini Palazzoli, M. *Self-Starvation. From the Intrapsychic to the Transpersonal Approach to Anorexia Nervosa.* London: Chaucer, 1974 (American ed.: New York, Jason Aronson, 1978).

Solyom, L., Freeman, R. J., & Miles, J. E. A comparative psychometric study of anorexia nervosa and obsessive neurosis. *Can. J. Psychiatry,* 27:282–286, 1982.

Solyom, J., Freeman, R. J., Thomas, C. D., & Miles, J. E. The comparative psychopathology of anorexia nervosa: Obsessive-compulsive disorder or phobia? *Internat. J. Eat. Dis.,* 3(1):3–14, 1983a.

Solyom, L., Thomas, C. D., Freeman, R. J., & Miles, J. E. Anorexia nervosa: Obsessive-compulsive disorder or phobia? A comparative study. In P. L. Darby, P. E. Garfinkel, D. M. Garner, & D. V. Coscina (Eds.), *Anorexia Nervosa: Recent Developments in Research.* New York: Alan R. Liss, 1983b, pp. 137–147.

Sours, J. *Starving to Death in a Sea of Objects. The Anorexia Nervosa Syndrome.* New York: Jason Aronson, 1980.

Szmukler, G. I. Drug treatment of anorexic states. In T. Silverstone (Ed.), *Drugs and Appetite.* London-New York: Academic Press, 1982, pp. 159–181.

Thomas, C. S. Dysmorphophobia: A question of definition. *Br. J. Psychiat.,* 144:513–516, 1984.

Trainor, D. MHP said responsive to pimozide therapy. *Psychiat. News,* August 1:5, 19, 1980.

Vandereycken, W. Neuroleptics in the short-term treatment of anorexia nervosa. A double-blind placebo-controlled study with sulpiride. *Br. J. Psychiatry,* 144:288–292, 1984.

Vandereycken, W., & Meermann, R. *Anorexia Nervosa. A Clinician's Guide to Treatment.* Berlin-New York: Walter de Gruyter, 1984.

Vandereycken, W., & Pierloot, R. Pimozide combined with behavior therapy in the short-term treatment of anorexia nervosa. A double-blind placebo-controlled cross-over study. *Acta Psychiat. Scand.,* 66:445–450, 1982.

Vandereycken, W., & Pierloot, R. Combining drugs and behavior therapy in anorexia nervosa: A double-blind placebo/pimozide study. In P. L. Darby, P. E. Garfinkel, D. M. Garner, & D. V. Coscina (Eds.), *Anorexia Nervosa: Recent Developments in Research.* New York: Alan R. Liss, 1983, pp. 365–375.

Van der Weyden, M. B., Collecutt, M. F., Davidson, A., & Faragher, B. S. Chlorpromazine-associated haemolysis in anorexia nervosa. *Acta Haematol.,* 73:111–113, 1985.

Volmat, R., Allers, G., Vittouris, N., & Dufay, F. Statut actuel clinique et thérapeutique de l'anorexie mentale. *Ann. Méd. Psychol.,* 128(2):161–184, 1970.

Weizman, R., Tyano, S., Wijsenbeek, H., & Ben David, M. Behavior therapy, pimozide treatment and prolactin secretion in anorexia nervosa. *Psychother. Psychosom.,* 43:136–140, 1985.

Zarr, M. L. Psychobiology of the borderline disorders—A heuristic approach. *Psychiat. Quart.,* 56:215–228, 1984.

5

Lithium in the Treatment of Eating Disorders

L. K. George Hsu

Lithium is a monovalent alkaline metal that occurs naturally as salts. Although present in minute quantities in animal tissue, it has no known physiological role. Cade (1949), while attempting to identify presumptive toxic nitrogenous substances in the urine of mental patients, gave lithium urate to guinea pigs and found that the animals became lethargic. In an inductive leap Cade then treated 19 agitated psychotic patients with lithium salts and reported that lithium seems to have rather specific antimanic effects. In the 1960s the effectiveness of lithium for the treatment of bipolar disorder became established in Europe and it was accepted for this use in the United States in 1970.

LITHIUM IN ANOREXIA NERVOSA

Medications have not proven to be particularly effective in the treatment of anorexia nervosa, either in the short term or in the long run (Hsu, 1986). Anecdotal case reports have found lithium to improve the mood disturbance in anorexia nervosa and also to produce weight gain (for review see Stein, Hartshorn, Jones, & Steinberg, 1982). All the cases reviewed by Stein et al. (1982) apparently belonged to the bulimic or vomiting subgroup of anorexia nervosa. To the best of my knowledge there exists only one double-blind controlled study of the use of lithium in treating anorexia nervosa. Gross, Ebert, Faden, Goldberg, et al. (1981) treated 16 female anorexia nervosa patients in a four-week double-blind lithium versus placebo study. All of the 16 patients also participated in an inpatient behavioral modification treatment program. Two significant findings emerged from a large number of variables analyzed: the lithium group showed greater weight gain at weeks three and four and the group also improved on the denial or minimization of illness item of the Psychiatric Rating Scale. Other measures such as the depression and obsessive-compulsive subscale of the Hopkins Symptom Checklist improved with treatment in both groups, but to a greater extent in the lithium group.

A major difficulty associated with evaluating the efficacy of medication in anorexia nervosa is finding the right outcome parameter to measure. More rapid weight gain within a specified time is unsatisfactory as an index of efficacy since it is not apparently correlated with better long-term outcome. If a medication is effective in treating anorexia nervosa, it would have to be able to prevent relapse, i.e., to maintain normal eating behavior and normal body weight over a period of months or years.

LITHIUM IN BULIMIA NERVOSA

No double-blind controlled studies exist in the use of lithium in treating bulimia nervosa. Hsu (1984) used lithium carbonate in an open trial involving 14 female bulimic patients; eight of these patients were given lithium concurrently with cognitive behavior therapy, whereas six patients were given lithium after cognitive therapy had failed. Twelve of the 14 patients showed marked (100% reduction in binge/purge episodes) or moderate (75% reduction) improvement. Follow-up at six to 16 months after the four- to eight-week course of lithium found most of the patients to have maintained their improvement. More recently the author has treated, in another six-week open trial, 17 patients with lithium in combination with some cognitive behavioral therapy (self-monitoring of intake, dietary instructions, and self-instructions when urges to binge occur). Eleven patients showed a marked or moderate improvement (at least 75% reduction), whereas six showed no improvement (less than 50% reduction in binge/purge episodes). The Eating Attitudes Test and Beck Depression Inventory scores decreased in almost all the patients regardless of whether their eating habits improved (Hsu, 1984). In the absence of a double-blind controlled trial, the effectiveness of lithium in bulimia nervosa must remain speculative.

Lithium used in conjunction with a tricyclic or a monoamine oxidase inhibitor is apparently effective in the treatment of otherwise refractory cases of depression (DeMontigny, Cournoyer, Morissette, Langlois, & Caille, 1983; Heninger, Charney, & Sternberg, 1983). I have given lithium to six bulimic patients who did not respond to adequate doses of a tricyclic or a monoamine oxidase inhibitor, and three of the patients improved within a week of the addition of lithium. These results must be regarded as very preliminary.

Again, simply using short-term outcome as a criterion for the efficacy of medication in treating bulimia nervosa may be problematic. Mitchell, Davis, and Goff (1985) reported a relapse rate of 40% within the first year in a series of 75 patients who had become abstinent for at least two months. Therefore, the efficacy of a medication in bulimia nervosa may have to be judged by its ability to prevent relapse.

SIDE EFFECTS OF LITHIUM

The side effects of lithium in eating disorders are potentially dangerous. Lithium toxicity may occur easily in a patient who is vomiting, abusing laxatives, abusing diuretics, and reducing fluid intake. In addition, cardiac abnormalities, which are common in cachectic patients, are likely to be exacerbated by lithium (Tilkian, Schroeder, Kao, & Huttgren, 1976). Thus, frequent (two times per week) monitoring of serum lithium levels and electrolytes is essential.

Side effects of lithium in anorexia nervosa have not been documented in detail. Neither Stein et al. (1982) nor Gross et al. (1981) reported on the side effects of lithium in the patients they treated. In the bulimic patients whom I have treated, side effects are uncommon if lithium level is kept at 0.6 to 0.8 meq/1 (see Practical Suggestions section). Nausea is the most common side effect and occurs in 20% of the patients. This side effect can be minimized by the patient's taking the lithium after a meal or by changing to a controlled release type of lithium. Itchiness and skin rash occurred in less than 10% of the patients. Changing the lithium to the liquid form of lithium citrate may help, but the patients usually find the taste of lithium citrate objectionable. Weight gain of over 10 pounds occurred in less than 10% of the patients, but it was unclear whether this occurred as a result of more normal eating and less vomiting or whether it was an effect of the lithium. Severe headache and blurred vision occurred in a patient with a previous history of migraine. Her lithium level was 1.1 meq/1, and subsequent reduction of the lithium dosage to maintain a lithium level at 0.6 to 0.8 meq/1 was not associated with a return of the headache. Thirst and increased urination occurred in two patients, which necessitated the termination of lithium. A year later one of these patients had a course of ECT for her major depression and she developed hypomanic features. She was again given lithium, and maintenance lithium has so far (one year) not been associated with the return of increased urination.

PRACTICAL SUGGESTIONS

In the absence of definitive evidence of the efficacy of lithium in the treatment of eating disorders, the use of lithium as the first line of treatment is not warranted. However, in patients who are resistant to other kinds of treatment, a trial of lithium may be worthwhile. It is my practice to give lithium in a single dose at bedtime, and for blood levels to be taken in the morning about 12 hours after this evening dose. For bulimic patients I have found that they respond well to a blood level of 0.6 to 0.8 meq/1, and increasing the blood level to beyond this range apparently does not confer any additional benefit. Patients maintained at this low therapeutic range rarely complain of side effects other than some initial nausea. It has also been my experience that lithium works best when combined with cognitive behavioral techniques. A double-blind trial of lithium versus placebo is currently underway.

POSSIBLE MECHANISMS OF ACTION

Why lithium may be effective in the treatment of eating disorders is not known. One possibility is that it acts by stabilizing mood disturbance. Certainly many bulimics report an increase in their urge to binge when they are depressed, and many complain of mood lability. Two studies have found that lithium may be effective in emotionally labile patients (Gram & Rafaelson, 1972; Rifkin, Quitkin, Carrillo, Blumberg, & Klein, 1972). Another possibility is that lithium may promote normal eating by its insulinlike action (Battacharya, 1964). The role of insulin in the regulation of eating and satiety has been the subject of much recent research (for a review, see Stricker, 1982). A third possibility is that lithium acts directly on the feeding center through its effect on the dopamine and/or opioid systems (Gillman & Lichtigfeld, 1985). These possible mechanisms are not mutually exclusive, but direct evidence to support any of them is still lacking.

REFERENCES

Battacharya, G. Influence of lithium and glucose metabolism in rats and rabbits. *Biochem. Biophys. Acta,* 93:644–646, 1964.

Cade, J.F.J. Lithium salts in the treatment of psychotic excitement. *Med. J. Australia,* 2:349-352, 1949.

DeMontigny, C., Cournoyer, G., Morissette, R., Langlois, R., & Caille, G. Lithium carbonate addition in tricyclic antidepressant-resistant unipolar depression. *Arch. Gen. Psychiatry,* 40:1327-1334, 1983.

Gillman, M. A., & Lichtigfeld, E. J. Lithium and bulimia: The role of the dopaminergic and opiatergic system. *Am. J. Psychiatry,* 142:1522-1523, 1985.

Gram, L. F., & Rafaelson, O. J. Lithium treatment of psychotic children and adolescents. *Acta Psychiat. Scand.,* 48:253-260, 1972.

Gross, H. A., Ebert, M. H., Faden, V. B., Goldberg, S. C., Lee, L. E., & Kaye, W. H. A double-blind controlled trial of lithium carbonate in primary anorexia nervosa. *J. Clin. Psychopharmacol.,* 1:376-381, 1981.

Heninger, G. R., Charney, D. S., & Sternberg, D. E. Lithium carbonate augmentation of antidepressant treatment. *Arch. Gen. Psychiatry,* 40:1335-1342, 1983.

Hsu, L.K.G. Treatment of bulimia with lithium. Unpublished manuscript, 1986.

Hsu, L.K.G. Treatment of bulimia with lithium. *Am. J. Psychiatry,* 141:1260-1262, 1984.

Mitchell, J. E., Davis, L., & Goff, G. The process of relapse in patients with bulimia. *Internat. J. Eat. Dis.,* 4:457-464, 1985.

Rifkin, A., Quitkin, F., Carrillo, C., Blumberg, A. G., & Klein, D. F. Lithium carbonate in emotionally unstable character disorder. *Arch. Gen. Psychiatry,* 27:519-523, 1972.

Stein, G. S., Hartshorn, J., Jones, J., & Steinberg, D. Lithium in a case of severe anorexia nervosa. *Br. J. Psychiatry,* 140:526-528, 1982.

Stricker, E. M. The central control of food intake: A role for insulin. In B. G. Hoebel & D. Novin (Eds.), *The Neural Basis of Feeding and Reward.* Brunswick: Haer Institute, 1982.

Tilkian, A. G., Schroeder, J. S., Kao, J., & Huttgren, H. The cardiovascular effects of lithium in mania. *Am. J. Med.,* 61:665-670, 1976.

6

Anticonvulsant Treatment of Eating Disorders

Allan S. Kaplan

Anorexia nervosa and bulimia nervosa remain puzzling disorders. Historically, etiologic thinking in both disorders has been characterized by dichotomous approaches. At various points in time, these disorders have been viewed as either totally psychologically determined or totally biologically based. Therapies for the eating disorders have reflected these viewpoints. Within the last 10 years, several authors have proposed a biopsychosocial model for understanding the eating disorders (Anderson, 1985; Garfinkel & Garner, 1982; Vandereycken & Meermann, 1984).

A significant body of research related to biologic therapies for anorexia nervosa and bulimia nervosa has focused on an apparent relationship between eating disorders and affective disorders (Cantwell, Sturzenberger, Burroughs, Salkin, & Green, 1977; Gwirtsman, Roy-Byrne, Yager, & Gerner, 1983; Hudson, Pope, & Jonas, 1983; Kaplan, Garfinkel, Warsh, & Brown, 1986; Piran, Kennedy, Garfinkel, & Owens, 1985; Pope, Hudson, Jonas, & Yurgelun-Todd, 1983; Walsh, Stewart, & Wright, 1982; Winokur, March, & Mendels, 1980). Another theoretical framework from which to view the possible biologic basis for eating disorders relates to hypothesized neurophysiologic abnormalities in subcortical areas of the brain that mediate feeding. These same areas may be involved in the regulation of mood, sleep, and other circadian rhythms. Much of this literature has focused on the anticonvulsant treatment of bulimic patients. This chapter describes theoretical issues relevant to anticonvulsant therapy and evaluates the existing literature that deals with the treatment of eating disorders with anticonvulsants. This review primarily focuses on the use of such drugs in treating patients with bulimic symptomatology; however, it also includes the small available literature on the treatment of patients with restricting anorexia nervosa.

ANOREXIA NERVOSA AND ANTICONVULSANTS

A possible rationale for treating anorexia nervosa patients with anticonvulsants relates to the small literature on EEG changes in such patients (Crisp, Fenton, & Scotton, 1968; Lundberg & Walinder, 1967; Nell, Merlkangus, Foster, et al., 1980). In one study, more than 60% of a group of patients with anorexia nervosa had EEG abnormalities (Crisp et al., 1968). In another study, Goor (1954) reported four anorexics with abnormal EEGs with similar findings in 11 of 15 family members. Although this suggests some genetic defect, these changes are almost always the result of complications of the illness and do not seem to be related to its etiology. In most instances, EEG changes most closely are related to disturbances in serum electrolytes, but might also reflect structural changes detected by computerized tomography (CT) in anorexia nervosa (Grebb, Yingling, & Reus, 1984). Convulsions are not uncommon in patients who have anorexia nervosa. Several studies have found that at least 10% of patients have convulsions (Crisp et al., 1968; Dalby, 1975). Once again, these probably reflect metabolic derangement and not inherent cortical irritability in patients who have anorexia nervosa.

There is little scientific evidence or theoretical rationale for treating patients with anorexia nervosa with anticonvulsants. There is one incredulous theory that proposes the illness is caused by a state of hypercortisolism (Sapse & Parsons, 1985). Available scientific evidence suggests that the hypercortisolism is not a cause of the illness but probably a result of weight loss (Doerr, Fichter, Pirke, & Lund, 1980). The proponents of a hypercortisolism theory propose treatment with cortisol antagonists, one of which is phenytoin. There have been no controlled studies on the use of phenytoin or any other anticonvulsant in anorexia nervosa, and its effectiveness at this point has no empirical or clinical support.

BULIMIA NERVOSA AND ANTICONVULSANTS

The occurrence of binge eating as a symptom in other medical conditions provides a possible clue to its etiology when it occurs as a separate syndrome without obvious organicity. However, although there is little doubt that for many patients disturbances in eating behavior are related to emotional factors, a small group of patients may have an underlying neurophysiologic basis for their bulimia nervosa. In the next section, a review of organic states in which bulimic behavior may occur leads to a discussion of the rationale for the use of anticonvulsants. This is followed by a review of treatment studies.

Bulimia Nervosa in Organic States

Animal Studies

The study of the pathophysiology of abnormal eating behavior in animals has focused primarily on the hypothalamus. Animal studies have shown that lesions in the ventromedial nucleus of the hypothalamus leads to hyperphagia (Hetherington & Ranson, 1940). Electrical stimulation of the lateral hypothalamic region causes a satiated animal to seek and consume food voraciously (Anand & Duw, 1955). The various brain amine systems also affect hunger and satiety. Catecholamines, specifically norepinephrine and dopamine, as well as indolamines, such as serotonin and its precursors, have marked effects on food intake when administered either intracerebrally, intravenously, or through diet (Garfinkel & Coscina, 1982). The exact effects of the neurotransmitters are not completely clear; what is clear is that they substantially influence hunger and satiety and feeding behavior in animals and probably humans and can, under certain circumstances, induce hyperphagia and weight gain.

Other endocrine and metabolic mechanisms seem to play a role in the regulation of eating. These include the levels of blood glucose and insulin, lipid stores, thermostatic controls, amino acid and protein intake, and gastroenteropancreatic variables, especially hormones. These mechanisms are not elaborated on further, other than to indicate that they point to the complexity of the physiologic control of hunger, satiety, and feeding behavior in both animals and probably in man.

Human Studies

a) Brain diseases

Considering the complexity of the mechanisms that affect feeding behavior, it is not surprising that bulimiclike behavior often accompanies various brain diseases in humans. Hyperphagia, increased aggressivity, and a dementialike picture can result from neoplasms in the ventromedial hypothalamic region (Reeves & Plum, 1969). The Klüver-Bucy syndrome, in which there is bilateral temporal lobe ablation, is characterized by visual agnosia, compulsive licking and biting, hypersexuality, and polyphagia (Terzian & Dalle Ore, 1955). Hyperphagia has been associated not only with neoplasms but also with other forms of brain lesions. It has been described in degenerative brain disorders such as Alzheimer's disease (Kirschbaum, 1951), in Huntington's chorea (Whittier, 1976), and in Parkinson's disease (Rosenberg, Herishanu, & Bellin, 1977). It occurs in postinfective neurologic conditions such as encephalitis and general paresis (Kirschbaum, 1951). It has also been reported following a variety of traumatic brain conditions, including frontal lobotomy or accidental damage to the frontal cortex (Hofstatter, Smolik, & Busch, 1945; Kirschbaum, 1951).

b) Bulimia nervosa as a form of seizure disorder

There is a literature suggesting that some forms of binge eating are the symptomatic manifestation of an underlying seizure disorder. Certain types of epilepsy, especially complex partial seizures, have a clear-cut temporal lobe focus and bulimic behavior is part of the postictal phenomena observed. Kleine-Levin syndrome, in which there is periodic hypersomnia and compulsive eating, usually in adolescent males, has been associated with well-documented mild or moderately diffuse EEG abnormalities (Wilkus & Chiles, 1975). Slowing of alpha rhythm while patients were symptomatic and a reversion to normal between attacks have been observed in this syndrome (Wilkus & Chiles, 1975). Stunkard, Grace, and Wolff (1955) allude to these phenomena in describing a series of obese bulimics whom they considered to have hypothalamic dysregulation. Such dysregulation could be the result of a subcortical irritability. Stunkard et al. (1955) classified these patients into night eaters and binge eaters. The night eater's behavior was considered to be consistent with a disturbance in the satiety center, whereas the binge eater's was suggestive of a disturbance in the appetite center of the hypothalamus. Moskovitz and Lingao (1979) reported binge eating associated with the oral contraceptive and abnormal EEGs.

Some investigators view the syndrome of bulimia nervosa as primarily a neurological disorder with epilepticlike characteristics (Rau & Green, 1975). Symptoms suggestive of this view consist of discrete episodic egodystonic compulsive eating episodes, usually preceded by auralike sensations. These sensations can include flashes of light, unusual smells, and increasing psychological tension prior to bingeing. Often such episodes are associated with mild depersonalization during the binge and sleepiness followed by disorientation and amnesia. Remick, Jones, & Campus (1980) have reported episodes of bulimia nervosa postictally in patients with temporal lobe EEG abnormalities. Pyle, Mitchell, and Eckert (1981) describe bulimia nervosa occurring with kleptomania and chemical abuse, and they suggest that these are indications of loss of generalized impulse control with a possible neurologic basis.

Bulimia nervosa that may be neurologically based has been described as being associated with certain diffuse neurologic soft signs and symptoms (Rau & Green, 1975). These include rage attacks that occur episodically, with no psychologic precipitant or pattern, the so-called episodic dyscontrol syndrome (Tunks & Dermer, 1977). Headaches, dizziness, gastrointestinal symptoms, paresthesias, perceptual disturbances such as depersonalization, derealization, déja vu, hypnogogic or hypnopompic hallucinations, and compulsive behaviors such as kleptomania are also reported.

Abnormal EEG patterns have been reported in patients with bulimia nervosa and without known seizure disorders. Rau and Green (1984) found 38 of 59 people with "binge eating syndrome" had abnormal EEGs. The most commonly found abnormality associated with binge eating is the 14- and six-per-second positive spiking pattern. There is controversy in the literature as to whether this is an abnormality or a variant of normal. The EEG pattern has a high prevalence within asymptomatic control populations, especially adolescence, where studies report the incidence to be anywhere from 25–58% (Wegner & Struve, 1977). The consensus in the literature is that this pattern is infrequent in the very young child, is increasingly prevalent in later childhood and in adolescence, and is rare in adulthood.

Gibbs and Gibbs (1965) have found the incidence of positive spiking in referred patients over the age of 29 to be 6%, or 20 times greater than the corresponding incidence among normal controls. In a study of the incidence of 14- and six-positive spiking in an adult psychiatric population age 30–39 compared to an asymptomatic adult control group, Wegner found 13% of the former as opposed to only 0.9% of the latter demonstrate this pattern. This represents a 15-fold increase in patient versus control sample. Interestingly, of the 42 nonhospitalized siblings of the patient group age 21–30,

16.7% displayed this EEG pattern, whereas only 6.5% of a control group in the age range displayed such a pattern. Studies have found symptoms of emotional instability, irritability, depression, rage along with a high probability of suicidal ideation, and gestures and attempts in association with this EEG pattern (Struve, Feighenbaum, & Farnum, 1972).

The importance of this 14- and six-positive spiking pattern lies in the fact that this occurs in 37% of the 59 bulimics in one particular study (Rau & Green, 1984) and accounted for almost 60% of the abnormal EEGs found in this group. This pattern was found to be the most reliable predictor of neurologic substrate for bulimia nervosa and of positive response to anticonvulsant therapy. However, other investigators (Mitchell, Hosfield, & Pyle, 1983; Wermuth, Davis, Hollister, & Stunkard, 1977) have not found this pattern in bulimic patients.

The present author, in his work with a series of 38 bulimic patients given cortical lead EEGs, found that three had identified seizure disorders which were reflected in clearly abnormal EEG patterns. Of the remaining 35 patients, only one had a questionable EEG pattern described as "instability during prolonged hyperventilation of the constitutional type." A subgroup of eight patients had nasopharyngeal EEGs, still with no abnormalities found.

There are difficulties in the interpretation of these data. One problem is that this EEG pattern almost always appears during drowsy and sleep states and not in the awake state (Gibbs & Gibbs, 1965). Awake EEGs will not usually detect this abnormality. Another difficulty relates to the fact that, as stated previously, some investigators regard this pattern as normal and, therefore, do not report it in their investigations. There is also a 40–50% false-negative probability in known grand mal epileptics in EEG reporting (Gibbs & Gibbs, 1965). A normal EEG does not exclude underlying brain abnormalities. Finally, rigorous diagnostic criteria for bulimia nervosa were not employed in these electroencephalographic studies, and this limits the generalizability of findings to patients with bulimia as a primary diagnosis.

In summary, the literature is not clear as to whether or not the 14- and six-per-second positive spiking is abnormal, is found more often among bulimic patients, or has any etiologic significance when it is present.

Studies of Anticonvulsant Treatment

A summary of studies of anticonvulsant treatment of bulimia nervosa is presented in Table 6-1.

Treatment with Phenytoin

a) Uncontrolled trials

Based on the theoretical perspective equating bulimia nervosa with a seizure disorder, Green and Rau (1974) initially reported on 10 patients with "compulsive eating disorder" treated openly with this drug. The following three diagnostic groups of patients were delineated: anorexia nervosa, normal weight patients who probably would have met the DSM-III criteria for bulimia nervosa and obese "compulsive eaters." Nine of the 10 patients had abnormal EEGs; six of the nine demonstrated the 14- and six-per-second positive spiking pattern. Four patients showed spiking in the temporal and occipital areas, and one patient had a normal EEG.

All patients were treated with phenytoin in an open trial. Nine of the 10 responded with cessation of bingeing. In further studies by the same investigators (Green and Rau, 1977), phenytoin was given to 26 patients with "compulsive eating." At a dosage of 400 mg given in an open trial, nine patients responded and 17 did not. Six of the 12 patients with abnormal EEGs and three of the 14 with normal EEGs responded to phenytoin with the cessation of bingeing. Of the 26 patients, seven were said to be "true compulsive eaters." Their bingeing was described as irregular, unpredictable, and egodystonic. Five of these seven patients had abnormal EEGs and six responded to dilantin. These seven patients described their binges as analogous to seizures, in that they were preceded by an inability

Table 6-1
Anticonvulsant Treatment of Bulimia Nervosa: Summary of Studies and Case Reports

Investigator(s)	Drug	Type of Study	Number of Subjects	EEG Pattern	Response
1. Green & Rau (1974)	phenytoin	uncontrolled	10	9 of 10 abnormal 6 had 14 + 6/sec spiking	9 of 10 stopped bingeing
2. Rau & Green (1975)	phenytoin	uncontrolled	26	12 abnormal 14 normal	6 responders 3 responders
3. Rau & Green (summary of studies to 1984)	phenytoin	uncontrolled	59	38 abnormal	27 responders 8 partial responders
4. Davis et al. (1974)	phenytoin	uncontrolled	5	4 abnormal	"general improvement"

5. Weiss & Levitz (1976)	phenytoin	uncontrolled	1	mildly abnormal	no response
6. Moore & Rakes (1982)	phenytoin	uncontrolled	1	14 + 6/sec spiking	response
7. Wermuth et al. (1977)	phenytoin	controlled	19	3 definitely abnormal 4 – 14 + 6/sec spiking	9 moderate or marked improvement
8. Greenway et al. (1977)	phenytoin	controlled	4 (obese)	1 questionably abnormal	no response as measured by weight loss and hunger ratings
9. Kaplan et al. (1983)	carbamazepine	controlled	6	normal	1 marked response
10. Kaplan et al. (1986)	carbamazepine	controlled	10	normal	1 moderate response 9 minimal or no response

to concentrate with depersonalization, detachment, and a postbinge phase of sleepiness and confusion. In a summary of their experience with phenytoin in the treatment of bulimia nervosa, Rau and Green (1984) reported that when 30 of 59 bulimic patients with abnormal EEGs and 17 of 21 bulimic patients with normal EEGs were treated openly, 70% of the patients with abnormal EEGs improved compared with 35% of those with normal EEGs, a significant difference. These same investigators suggest that phenytoin response was more likely to occur in subjects whose weight deviated by 25% or more from normal.

Other investigators have reported on the use of phenytoin in single cases. Weiss and Levitz (1976) describe a bulimic patient with a past history of anorexia nervosa who showed no response to therapeutic doses of dilantin despite the fact that her EEG was mildly abnormal and similar to those of patients described by Green and Rau. In contrast, Moore and Rakes (1982) report one case in which the patient had periodic, very distinct episodes of bulimia characterized by acute onsets, well demarcated endings lasting four to six weeks, with normal eating in between episodes. Her EEG during a binge episode revealed 14- and six-per-second positive spiking in the right temporal and occipital areas. Treatment with phenytoin led to remission for one year while on the drug, relapse when the drug was discontinued, and remission again when the drug was reinstated. Davis, Quallis, Hollister, and Stunkard (1974) report on five patients who probably fulfilled the DSM-III criteria. All were between the ages of 21 and 53 with no history of a seizure disorder in themselves or their families. Four demonstrated significant EEG abnormalities on sleep-deprived nasopharyngeal lead recordings; two had bilateral independent antero-medial temporal spikes; one showed six-per-second spiking and slow wave frontal region waves. These findings led the authors to conduct a controlled treatment trial, described later in this chapter (Wermuth et al., 1977). Finally, Pope and Hudson (1984) report treating 10 bulimics with phenytoin with only one patient reporting a modest reduction in urge to binge but with continued improvement once the drug was stopped.

b) Controlled trials

There have been few controlled studies of phenytoin in bulimia nervosa. Wermuth et al. (1977) conducted a 12-week double-blind trial and found phenytoin to be considerably less effective than previously reported. In the phenytoin-placebo group, five of 10 patients were moderately to markedly improved; three showed no change compared to placebo. In the placebo-phenytoin group, four showed marked to moderate improvement, whereas three showed slight and two no improvement. Interestingly, there was a persistence of treatment effect in the placebo period after initial treatment with phenytoin. Definite abnormal EEGs were seen in three subjects and four others had the 14- and six-positive-per-second spiking. EEG abnormalities were not correlated with treatment response. A shorter duration of bingeing was correlated with a positive response, whereas a history of anorexia nervosa was associated with no response.

Greenway, Dahms, and Bray (1977) studied the use of phenytoin in obese "compulsive eaters." Their primary interest was in the efficacy of the drug in inducing weight loss. Ninety-eight (98) obese patients were given a questionnaire to detect compulsive eating behaviors. This questionnaire asked the following five questions: (1) What percent of the time do you think about food? (2) Do you crave food? (3) Do you get up during the night to eat? (4) Do you find yourself eating more food shortly after finishing a large meal? (5) Do you eat large quantities of food in short periods of time even when not hungry? Four of the highest-scoring subjects were then treated with phenytoin and placebo in a double-blind crossover study. All patients had normal EEGs. Phenytoin was ineffective in producing weight loss or in changing subjective hunger ratings compared to placebo. Actual number of binges was not reported.

There are several problems with this study. Only the last question specifically refers to bulimic behavior; it is doubtful that patients in this study scoring high on the questionnaire would actually fulfill DSM-III criteria for bulimia nervosa. The number of binges was not measured, and the dependent variable by which drug efficacy was measured was weight.

Generally, serious methodologic flaws are evident in the studies with phenytoin. Sample sizes have been too small to allow sophisticated data analysis that would yield information related to characteristics of responders versus nonresponders. The duration of follow-up periods has been inadequate. Criteria for bulimia nervosa have not been uniform; there have been too few properly controlled trials. The evidence at this point suggesting that bulimia nervosa is a form of a seizure disorder that responds to phenytoin therapy comes from only one group of investigators whose findings have not been replicated by others.

Treatment with Carbamazepine

Carbamazepine appears to have therapeutic effects on mood and behavior that have some organic basis. Theoretically, it bridges both pathophysiologic models of conceptualizing bulimia nervosa; that is, its relationship to affective disorders and seizure disorders. To help further understand its effectiveness in these conditions, Post and Kopanda (1976) have postulated a kindling model of psychopathology. According to this model, accumulative bioelectric changes in the limbic area are secondary to repeated psychological or biochemical stresses leading to abnormal limbic neuronal activity and eventual psychiatric disturbances. Carbamazepine's mechanism of action in conditions in which it is effective appears related to subcortical and more preferential limbic activity. It has the unique ability to preferentially depress transmission across polysynaptic pathways into and from limbic nuclei (Hernandez-Peon, 1964).

Another separate but interesting possible mechanism for considering carbamazepine in treating bulimia nervosa is its effect on neurotransmitters such as indoleamines. Reynolds (1984) has shown that carbamazepine elevates whole and free tryptophan levels, possibly through its effect on inhibiting liver tryptophan pyrrolase (Badawy & Evans, 1981). This would lead to a rise in central serotonin, theoretically affecting mood as well as satiety mechanisms.

Such effects on the limbic system and on serotonin and other neurotransmitters could explain carbamazepine's proven efficacy in treating conditions that have been associated with bulimia nervosa, such as behavioral disorders associated with epilepsy, affective disorders, and alcoholism.

a) Use in related conditions

In over 40 reports involving some 2,500 patients, carbamazepine has been found in about 50% of cases to exhibit a positive psychotropic effect on the behavioral disorders occurring in epileptic patients (Dalby, 1975). Most of these studies were uncontrolled clinical trials, although seven were double-blind placebo-controlled trials. This effect leads to positive affective changes, especially reduced anxiety and depression and to improvement in intellectual capacities, increased drive and initiative, social behavior, and lessened impulsivity.

Nonepileptic behaviorally disturbed patients with nonspecific EEG abnormalities also have improved on carbamazepine as compared to placebo (Groh, 1976). Symptoms that were most improved were disturbances in drive, dysphoria, and anxiety. Puente (1976) demonstrated significant clinical improvement with carbamazepine compared to placebo in a group of behaviorally disturbed children with cerebral dysfunction. Kuhn (1976) showed that a majority of behaviorally disturbed children studied responded to carbamazepine; many of these had a family history of significant mental illness. Tunks and Dermer (1977) illustrated the usefulness of carbamazepine in treating adult patients who have the so-called "dyscontrol syndrome." Gardner and Cowdry (1986) demonstrated the efficacy of carbamazepine in controlling impulsive behavior in a group of borderline patients. Reid, Naylor, and Kay (1981) in a double-blind placebo-controlled crossover trial of carbamazepine showed that in a group of profoundly mentally retarded overactive adults there was a significant response to the drug. This was especially so in patients in whom overactivity was accompanied by elevation of mood.

According to Remschmidt (1976), "beneficial clinical results have been achieved with carbamazepine in the following target symptoms more or less irrespective of their origin: hyperactivity, hyperkinesia and hypokinesia, lack of concentration, behavioral disturbances marked by aggressiveness, and mood disorders of a dysphoric type" (p. 253).

Carbamazepine has also been shown to be effective in treating affective disorders. Even before the first Japanese studies demonstrated the beneficial effect of carbamazepine on manic symptomatology, there were reports of its being therapeutic for treating manic or depressive states in epileptic patients or for atypical manic depressive psychosis (Cereghino, Brock, VanMeter, Penny, et al., 1974; Mystener, 1968). Okuma, Kishimoto, Inoue, Matsumoto, et al. (1973) obtained successful results with carbamazepine in the treatment of 18 out of 33 and in the prophylaxis of 13 of 27 manic patients. On a further 90 patients (Okuma & Kishimoto, 1977), carbamazepine was shown to have an antimanic effect in over half of the manic episodes and an antidepressant effect in one-third of depressive episodes. In two-thirds of cases it had a prophylactic effect against mania or depression. Okuma, Inanaga, Otsuki, Sarai, et al. (1979) showed that carbamazepine and chlorpromazine were equally effective in treating acute mania, with carbamazepine having significantly fewer side effects. Takezaki and Hanaoka (1971) found that psychosis occurring as part of a bipolar illness responded better (nine of 10 patients) than what they called symptomatic psychosis (four of 10 patients).

In the first double-blind placebo-controlled study of carbamazepine's efficacy in manic-depressive illness, Ballenger and Post (1980) found that half of 26 depressed patients showed evidence of antidepressant response, and seven of 12 manic patients showed antimanic response. Four manic patients had major relapses when placebo was substituted and improvement when carbamazepine was reinstituted. Carbamazepine prophylaxis was seen in nine patients, all of whom were not well controlled on lithium carbonate. In a study of the long-term prophylactic effects of carbamazepine in affective disorders (Kishimoto, Obura, Hazama, & Inoue, 1983), complete inhibition of manic and depressive episodes was observed in four of 32 cases with a reduced incidence of episodes and decreased intensity of symptoms in 20 of 32 patients. More recently, Post, Uhde, Roy-Byrne, and Joffe (1986) demonstrated acute antidepressant action of carbamazepine in about 60% of 35 depressed patients treated in a double-blind placebo-controlled study.

Carbamazepine has also been found to be effective in the treatment of alcohol withdrawal states (Bjorkquist, Isohanni, Makela, & Malinen, 1976), as well as in the treatment of other forms of paroxysmal disorders, such as the Klüver-Bucy syndrome (Hooshmand, Sepdham, & Vries, 1974).

b) Use in bulimia nervosa

The rationale for considering carbamazepine for bulimia nervosa relates to its effectiveness in the treatment of phasic epileptic disorders resembling functional psychiatric syndromes as well as other paroxysmal states. Carbamazepine has shown promise in the treatment of affective disorders. These conditions have been hypothesized to be etiologically related to subcortical dysregulation. As described previously, the pathophysiology of abnormal eating states in both animals and humans has focused on possible subcortical dysregulation in structures such as the hypothalamus. Bulimia nervosa may then be another condition for which carbamazepine is potentially useful.

Over the past five years, our group has been conducting a double-blind, placebo-controlled trial of carbamazepine in the treatment of bulimia nervosa (Kaplan et al., unpublished data). In a preliminary report (Kaplan, Garfinkel, Darby, & Garner, 1983) of the first six patients to complete this study, one experienced a complete remission with the drug and relapse on the placebo. The others had either minimal or no response.

In all, 16 patients have completed the study. All patients fit the DSM-III criteria for bulimia nervosa plus the frequency criterion of at least one binge per week with no binge-free intervals of longer than three weeks during the previous year. All patients gave informed written consent to the study. Patients were excluded from this study if they had documented clinical evidence of a major seizure disorder requiring the use of anticonvulsant medication in the year prior to the start of the investigation. Pregnant or nursing females and patients with a significant hepatic, hematologic, or coronary artery disease were also excluded from the study. Patients with a previous history of affective disorder were not excluded.

Following the initial assessment, the patient underwent baseline laboratory investigation, including CBC, liver function tests, electrolytes, urinalysis, thyroid indices, EKG, EEG, and a urine test for pregnancy. For a baseline period of two weeks the patients kept a record of the number of binges, number of purges, and a 10cm analogue scale of mood and a sense of control. Baseline and periodic psychometric testing included self-report instruments measuring a range of attitudinal, affective, and symptom dimensions.

Following the baseline, patients were placed in a double-blind crossover study. The first six patients were treated at six-week intervals over 18 weeks with placebo or carbamazepine in a placebo-carbamazepine-placebo or carbamazepine-placebo-carbamazepine double blind design. The next 10 patients were treated in two six-week intervals of placebo-carbamazepine or carbamazepine-placebo over 12 weeks. (The initial design was believed to be too lengthy and was leading to an excessive number of dropouts.)

All patients were seen weekly by the author. During this visit, patients received support and education that was related to their eating disorder, as well as a prescription for the following week's medication. Interpretive psychotherapy or cognitive restructuring was not part of the therapeutic contact. Patients underwent periodic blood tests, including serum levels of carbamazepine, the results of which were sent to another investigator, who then directed the primary one to either raise or lower the dose. This was done during both placebo and medication periods to maintain the double-blind design. Dosage was adjusted to maintain blood levels in the upper therapeutic range. Patients continued to monitor their eating behavior and mood throughout the study.

Figures 6-1 and 6-2 show individual patients' responses to carbamazepine. In the drug-placebo sequence (Figure 6-1), patient #4 and patient #8 demonstrated a reduction in binges compared to baseline, with patient #4 showing a more marked effect. There was no difference in the response to the drug compared to placebo. This

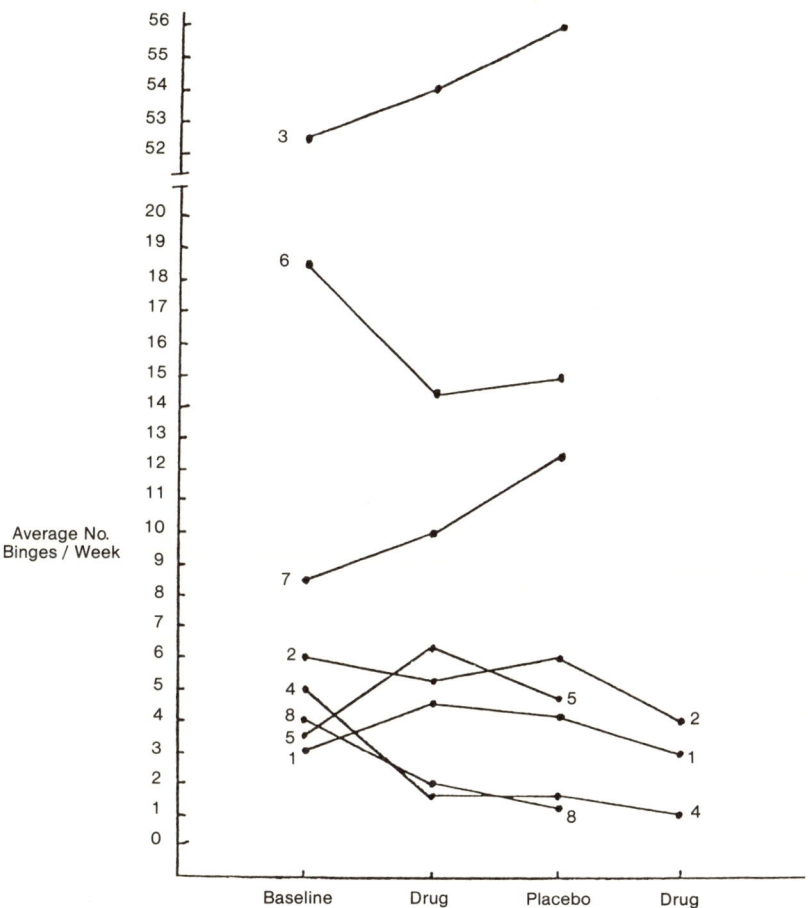

Figure 6-1. Bulimic response to carbamazepine (drug-placebo sequence).

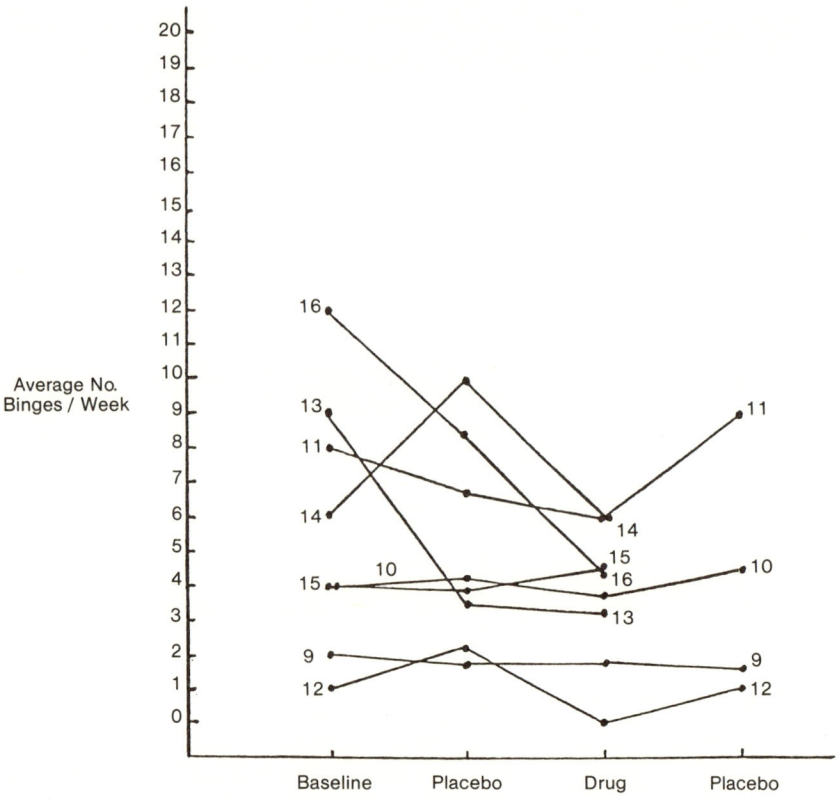

Figure 6-2. Bulimic response to carbamazepine (placebo-drug sequence).

can be partially explained by what has been reported in previous studies (Wermuth et al., 1977) where there appears to be an unexpected persistence of treatment effects in a placebo period for subjects in a drug placebo sequence. This is unlikely to be the result of a drug effect and more likely a behavioral or learning effect once the vicious cycle of bingeing and purging is interrupted.

In the placebo-drug sequence (Figure 6-2), patient #12, as previously reported (Kaplan et al., 1983), demonstrated remission during the drug period with relapse in the first and second placebo periods. Patient #16 demonstrated a slight decrease in bingeing in the drug period compared to placebo, and a more marked decrease in drug compared to baseline period. Patient #13 demonstrated decreased bingeing on both the drug and placebo compared to baseline. The explanation for this is most likely related to the effect of self-monitoring behavior that has been known to decrease bingeing (Johnson & Larson, 1982). Other nonspecific factors, such as the effect of weekly supportive contact or the illness entering a more restricting phase postbaseline, are plausible but unlikely explanations.

To summarize the results, of the 16 subjects treated, one (#12) had complete remission, and another (#16) a clear decrease in bingeing comparing drug to placebo periods. Three others (#4, #8, and #13) showed greater or less improvement comparing drug to baseline but no change comparing drug to placebo periods. Clinically, four of the five patients (#8 excepted) showed improvement with less depressed mood, increased socialization, and functioning with increased feeling of well-being. However, carbamazepine was not dramatically effective for the majority of patients who fulfilled DSM-III criteria for bulimia nervosa in this study. From the available evidence on the treatment of bulimia nervosa with phenytoin, the same seems to be true. There may be a small minority of bulimic patients who respond positively to one or both of these drugs. Further analysis of this study, correlating neuroendocrine and psychometric data with drug response, may offer some direction as to distinguishing such patients from a larger group of bulimics.

Combination of Seizure Disorders and Eating Disorders

The concomitant occurrence of eating disorders with other medical conditions can lead to difficult diagnostic as well as therapeutic challenges. There have been reports in the literature of diabetes and bulimia nervosa occurring in a higher than expected frequency and leading to difficult management problems (Hudson, Hudson, & Wentworth, 1983; Rodin, Daneman, Johnson, Kenshole, et al., 1986; Szmukler and Russell, 1983). Similarly, a small group of patients have a clearly documented seizure disorder as well as a well-defined eating disorder. It is not known whether the presence of a seizure disorder increases the risk of an eating disorder; epidemiologic studies in epileptic populations have not been done.

Nevertheless, this group of patients presents a formidable challenge for management. Adequate seizure control is often interfered with by the features of the eating disorder. Purging often leads to erratic blood levels of anticonvulsant medication. The seizure threshold can be lowered by an emaciated state or by metabolic alterations such as hypokalemia or hypoglycemia. During the course of the treatment of an eating disorder, medications such as antidepressants or phenothiazines are required and these drugs lower the seizure threshold, which can induce an epileptic attack. Conversely, the seizure disorder can interfere with a clearer understanding of the eating disorder. Patients can attribute their inability to control their eating to an underlying epileptic diathesis and in the process further confuse whether adjustments in treatment are needed for the eating disorder, the seizure disorder, or both.

The author has consulted on, or been involved in, the treatment of four patients who presented with seizure disorders and bulimia nervosa. In three of the cases, there were clearly documented EEG abnormalities and histories consistent with a diagnosis of a seizure disorder. In one case there was a previous history of a clear seizure disorder with a more recent onset of what sounded like pseudoseizures as opposed to true epileptic attacks. In two of the three other cases, the seizure disorder clearly preceded the eating disorder. The etiology of the epilepsy in two of these clearly documented cases was idiopathic. The third case was that of Sturge-Weber's Syndrome. This patient had been treated for several years with carbamazepine prior to the onset of her eating disorder and developed bulimia nervosa while she was on the drug.

Two subjects stopped bingeing in response to antidepressant drugs; however, the antidepressants (trazadone and amitryptiline) lowered the seizure threshold and led to poor seizure control. Constant monitoring of anticonvulsant medication is required in such cases to ensure adequate blood levels and seizure control. The use of newer generation nontricyclic antidepressant drugs for the management of such patients should be considered with the exception of maprotiline, which has been reported to induce seizures (Hollister, 1981). In all three documented cases, there appeared to be no obvious etiologic relationship between the seizure disorder and the eating disorder, but this could not be conclusively proven.

SUMMARY

Core-eating related symptomatology for the large majority of patients with anorexia nervosa and bulimia nervosa is not significantly altered by phenytoin or carbamazepine therapy, the two anticonvulsants that have been studied. A concomitant mood disturbance could theoretically respond to carbamazepine's proven thymoleptic action and may indirectly lead to improvement in other symptomatology, but this has not been rigorously studied. Combination of an eating disorder and seizure disorder requires skillful and careful management, with a working knowledge of psychotropic anticonvulsant drug interactions.

There is value in viewing bulimia nervosa from a model other than that which sees it as related to the affective disorders. Such alternate viewpoints, although more theoretically as opposed to empirically based, could potentially lead to greater understanding of the pathophysiology of this heterogeneous syndrome and in the process begin to focus subgroups of bulimic patients who are definably different on a number of parameters. Improved and more efficacious treatment, although still elusive, may ultimately result.

REFERENCES

Anderson, G. H. *Practical Comprehension Treatment of Anorexia Nervosa and Bulimia.* Baltimore, MD: John Hopkins University Press, 1985.

Anand, B. K., & Duw, S. Feeding responses induced by electrical stimulation of the hypothalamus in cat. *Indian J. Med. Res.,* 43:113–122, 1955.

Badawy, A. A., & Evans, M. Inhibition of rat liver tryptophan pyrrolase activity and elevation of brain tryptophan concentration by administration of antidepressants. *Biochem. Pharmacol.,* 30(11):1211–1216, 1981.

Ballenger, J. C., & Post, R. M. Carbamazepine in manic-depressive illness: A new treatment. *Am. J. Psychiatry,* 137(7):782–790, 1980.

Bjorkquist, S. E., Isohanni, B., Makela, R., & Malinen, L. Ambulant treatment of alcohol withdrawal symptoms with carbamazepine: A formal multicentre double-blind comparison with placebo. *Acta Psychiat. Scand.,* 53:333–342, 1976.

Cantwell, D. P., Sturzenberger, S., Burroughs, J., Salkin, B., & Green, J. K. Anorexia nervosa: An affective disorder? *Arch. Gen. Psychiatry,* 34:1087–1093, 1977.

Cereghino, J. J., Brock, J. T., VanMeter, J. C., Penny, J. K., Smith, L. D., & White, B. G. Carbamazepine for epilepsy: A controlled prospective evaluation. *Neurology,* 24:401–410, 1974.

Crisp, A. H., Fenton, G. W., & Scotton, L. A controlled study of the EEG in anorexia nervosa. *Br. J. Psychiatry,* 114:1149–1160, 1968.

Dalby, M. Behavioral effects of carbamazepine. In J. K. Penny & D. D. Daly (Eds.), *Advances in Neurology,* vol. II. New York: Raven Press, 1975.

Dally, P. *Anorexia Nervosa.* New York: Grune and Stratton, 1969.

Davis, K. L., Quallis, B., Hollister, L. E., & Stunkard, A. J. (Letter) EEGs of binge eaters. *Am. J. Psychiatry,* 131:1409, 1974.

Doerr, P., Fichter, M., Pirke, K. M., & Lund, R. (Abstract). Relationship between weight gain and hypothalamic-pituitary-adrenal function in patients with anorexia nervosa. Paper presented at Sixth International Congress of Endocrinology, Melbourne, Australia, 1980.

Gardner, D. L., & Cowdry, R. W. Positive effects of carbamazepine on behavioral dyscontrol in borderline personality disorder. *Am. J. Psychiatry,* 143:519–522, 1986.

Garfinkel, P. E., & Coscina, D. V. The physiology and psychology of hunger and satiety. In M. Fales (Ed.), *Eating, Sleeping, and Sexuality: Treatment of Disorders in Basic Life Functions.* New York: Brunner/Mazel, 1982, pp. 5–42.

Garfinkel, P. E., & Garner, D. M. *Anorexia Nervosa: A Multidimensional Perspective.* New York: Brunner/Mazel, 1982.

Gibbs, F. A., & Gibbs, E. L. Atlas of Electroencephalography, vol. 3. *Neurological and Psychiatric Disorders.* Reading, MA: Addison-Wesley, 1965.

Goor, E. EEG in anorexia nervosa. *Br. J. Psychiatry,* 6:349–351, 1954.

Grebb, J. A., Yingling, C. D., & Reus, V. I. Electrophysiologic abnormalities in patients with eating disorders. *Comprehen. Psychiatry,* 25(2):216–224, 1984.

Green, R. S., & Rau, J. J. Treatment of impulsive eating disturbances with anticonvulsant medication. *Am. J. Psychiatry,* 131:428–432, 1974.

Green, R. S., & Rau, J. H. The use of diphenylhydantoin in compulsive eating disorders: Further studies. In R. A. Vigersky (Ed.), *Anorexia Nervosa.* New York: Raven Press, 1977.

Greenway, F. L., Dahms, W. T., & Bray, G. A. Phenytoin as a treatment of obesity associated with compulsive eating. *Curr. Therap. Res.,* 21:338–342, 1977.

Groh, C. The psychotropic effect of Tegretol in non-epileptic children. In W. Birkmeyer (Ed.), *Epileptic Seizures-Behavior-Pain.* Vienna: Hans Huber, 1976, pp. 259–263.

Gwirtsman, H. E., Roy-Byrne, P., Yager, J., & Gerner, R. H. Neuroendocrine abnormalities in bulimia. *Am. J. Psychiatry,* 140:559–563, 1983.

Hernandez-Peon, R. Anticonvulsive action of G32883. *Neuropsychopharmacol.,* 3:303–311, 1964.

Hetherington, A. W., & Ranson, S. W. Hypothalamic lesions and adiposity in the rat. *Anat. Rec.,* 78:149, 1940.

Hofstatter, L., Smolik, E. A., & Busch, A. K. Prefrontal lobotomy in the treatment of chronic psychosis. *Arch. Neurol. (Chicago),* 53:125–130, 1945.

Hollister, L. E. Second generation antidepressant drugs. *Psychosomatics,* 22(10):872–879, 1981.

Hooshmand, H., Sepdham, T., & Vries, J. K. Klüver-Bucy Syndrome: Successful treatment with carbamazepine. *JAMA,* 229:1782, 1974.

Hudson, J. I., Pope, H. G., & Jonas, J. M. Phenomenologic relationship of eating disorders to major affective disorders. *Psychiat. Res.,* 9:345–354, 1983.

Hudson, J. I., Pope, H. G., Jonas, J. M., Laffer, P. S., Hudson, M. S., &

Melby, J. C. Hypothalamic-pituitary-adrenal axis hyperactivity in bulimia. *Psychiat. Res.,* 8:111–117, 1983.

Hudson, J. I., Pope, H. G., Jonas, J. M., & Yurgelun-Todd, D. Family history study of anorexia nervosa and bulimia. *Br. J. Psychiatry,* 142:133–138, 1983.

Hudson, M. S., Hudson, J. I., & Wentworth, S. M. Bulimia and diabetes. *New Eng. J. Med.,* 309:431–432, 1983.

Johnson, C., & Larson, R. Bulimia: An analysis of moods and behavior. *Psychosom. Med.,* 44(4):341–351, 1982.

Kaplan, A. S., Garfinkel, P. E., Darby, P. L., & Garner, D. M. Carbamazepine in the treatment of bulimia. *Am. J. Psychiatry,* 140:1225–1227, 1983.

Kaplan, A. S., Garfinkel, P. E., Warsh, J. J., & Brown, G. M. Neuroendocrine responses in bulimia. In *Proceedings of Disorders of Eating Behavior, Advances in Biosciences.* Oxford, England: Pergamon Press, 1986, pp. 241–245.

Kirschbaum, W. R. Excessive hunger as a symptom of cerebral origin. *J. Nerv. Ment. Dis.,* 113:95–114, 1951.

Kishimoto, A., Obura, C., Hazama, H., & Inoue, K. Long-term prophylactic effects of carbamazepine in affective disorder. *Br. J. Psychiatry,* 143:327–331, 1983.

Kuhn, R. The psychotropic effect of carbamazepine in non-epileptic adults, with particular reference to the drug's possible mechanism of action. In W. Birkmeyer (Ed.), *Epileptic Seizures-Behaviour-Pain.* Vienna: Hans Huber, 1976, pp. 264–267.

Lundberg, O., & Walinder, J. Anorexia nervosa and signs of brain damage. *Int. J. Neuropsychiat.,* 3:165–173, 1967.

Lutz, E. G. Alternative drug treatments in Gilles de la Tourette's Syndrome. *Am. J. Psychiatry,* 134:98–99, 1977.

Mitchell, J. E., Hosfield, W., & Pyle, R. EEG findings in patients with the bulimia syndrome. *Int. J. Eat. Disord.,* 2(3):17–21, 1983.

Moore, P. C. Amitryptiline therapy in anorexia nervosa. *Am. J. Psychiatry,* 134:1303–1304, 1977.

Moore, S. L., & Rakes, S. M. Binge-eating—Therapeutic response to dephenylhydantoin: Case report. *J. Clin. Psychiatry,* 43(9):385–386, 1982.

Moskovitz, R. A., & Lingao, A. Binge eating associated with oral contraceptives. *Am. J. Psychiatry,* 136(5):721–722, 1979.

Mystener, A. Carbamazepine treatment of epileptic psychosis. *Nord. Psychiat. Tidski,* 22:52–63, 1968.

Needleman, H. L., & Waber, D. The use of amitryptiline in anorexia nervosa. In R. A. Vigersky (Ed.), *Anorexia Nervosa.* New York: Raven Press, 1977, pp. 357–362.

Nell, J. F., Merlkangus, J. R., Foster, F. G., et al. Waking and all night sleep EEG's in anorexia nervosa. *Clin. Electroenc.,* 11:9–15, 1980.

Okuma, T., Kishimoto, A., Inoue, H., Matsumoto, H., Ogura, A., Matsushita, T., Nakao, T., & Ogura, C. Antimanic and prophylactic effects of carbamazepine (Tegretol) in manic depressive psychosis. *Folia Psychiat. Neurol.* (Japan), 27:283–297, 1973.

Okuma, T., & Kishimoto, A. (Abstract). Antimanic and prophylactic effects of Tegretol. Paper presented at the VIth World Congress of Psychiatry, Honolulu, Hawaii, 1977.

Okuma, T., Inanaga, S., Otsuki, K., Sarai, R., Takahashi, H., Hazama, A., Mori, A., & Watanabe, M. Comparison of the antimanic efficacy of carbamazepine and chlorpromazepine: A double-blind controlled study. *Psychopharmacol.,* 66:211–217, 1979.

Piran, N., Kennedy, S., Garfinkel, P. E., & Owens, M. Affective disturbance in eating disorders. *J. Nerv. Ment. Dis.,* 173(7):395–400, 1985.

Pope, H. G., Hudson, J. I., Jonas, J. M., & Yurgelun-Todd, D. Bulimia treated with imipramine: A placebo controlled, double-blind study. *Am. J. Psychiatry,* 140:554–558, 1983.

Pope, H. G., & Hudson, J. I. *New Hope for Binge Eaters.* New York: Harper & Row, 1984, p. 138.

Post, R. M., & Kopanda, P. P. Cocaine, kindling and psychosis. *Am. J. Psychiatry,* 133:6, 1976.

Post, R. M., Uhde, T. W., Roy-Byrne, P. P., & Joffe, R. T. Antidepressant effects of carbamazepine. *Am. J. Psychiatry,* 143(1):29–34, 1986.

Puente, R. M. The use of carbamazepine in the treatment of behavioral disorders in children. In W. Birkmeyer (Ed.), *Epileptic Seizures-Behaviour-Pain.* Vienna: Hans Huber, 1976, pp. 243–247.

Pyle, R. L., Mitchell, J. E., & Eckert, E. D. Bulimia: A report of 34 cases. *J. Clin. Psychiat.,* 42(2):60–64, 1981.

Rau, J. H., & Green, R. S. Binge-purge syndrome. Neurological factors affecting binge eating: Body over mind. In R. G. Hawkins, W. J.

Fremouw, & P. F. Clement (Eds.), *Diagnosis, Treatment and Research.* New York: Springer, 1984, pp. 123-143.

Rau, J. H., & Green, R. S. Compulsive eating: A neuropsychologic approach to certain eating disorders. *Comprehen. Psychiatry,* 16:223-231, 1975.

Reeves, A. G., & Plum, F. Hyperphagia, rage and dementia accompanying a ventromedial hypothalamic neoplasm. *Arch. Neurol.,* 20:616-624, 1969.

Reid, A., Naylor, G., & Kay, D. A double-blind placebo-conrolled crossover trial of carbamazepine in overactive severely mentally handicapped patients. *Psychol. Med.,* 11:109-113, 1981.

Remick, R. A., Jones, M. W., & Campus, P. E. Postictal bulimia. (Letter) *J. Clin. Psychiatry,* 41(7):256, 1980.

Remschmidt, H. The psychotropic effect of carbamazepine in nonepileptic patients, with particular reference to problems posed by clinical studies in children with behavioral disorders. In W. Birkmeyer (Ed.), *Epileptic Seizures-Behaviour-Pain.* Vienna: Hans Huber, 1976, pp. 253-258.

Reynolds, E. H. Temporal lobe epilepsy, behavior and anticonvulsant drugs. In M. E. Tremble and E. Zarifian (Eds.), *Psychopharmacology of the Lumber System.* Oxford, England: Oxford University Press, 1984.

Rodin, G., Daneman, D., Johnson, L., Kenshole, A., & Garfinkel, P. E. Eating disorders in female adolescents with insulin dependent diabetes mellitus. *Int. J. Psychiatry Med.,* 16:49-58, 1986.

Rompel, H., & Baumeister, P. W. Etiology of migraine and prevention with carbamazepine (Tegretol): Results of a double-blind, crossover study. *S.S. Afr. Med.,* 44:75-80, 1970.

Rosenberg, P., Herishanu, Y., & Bellin, B. Increased appetite (bulimia) in Parkinson's Disease. *Am. Geriat. Soc.,* 25(6):277-278, 1977.

Sapse, A. T., & Parsons, J. M. Cortisol: Cortisol receptors and anorexia nervosa. Paper presented at Eighth World Congress, Int. College of Psychosom. Med., Chicago, September, 1985.

Struve, F. A., Feighenbaum, Z. S., & Farnum, C. Prediction of 14 and 6-per-second positive spikes in EEGs of psychiatric patients. *Clin. Electroencephalogr.,* 3:60-64, 1972.

Stunkard, A. J., Grace, W. J., & Wolff, H. G. The nighteating syndrome: A pattern of food intake among certain obese patients. *Am. J. Med.,* 19:78, 1955.

Szmukler, G. I., & Russell, G. F. M. Diabetes mellitus, anorexia nervosa and bulimia. *Br. J. Psychiatry,* 142:305-308, 1983.

Takezaki, H., & Hanaoka, M. The use of carbamazepine in the control of manic-depressive psychosis and other manic states. *Clin. Psychiat.,* 13:173-183, 1971.

Terzian, A., & Dalle Ore, G. Syndrome of Kluver and Bucy reproduced in man by bilateral removal of the temporal lobes. *Neurol.,* 5:373, 1955.

Tunks, E. R., & Dermer, S. W. Carbamazepine in the dyscontrol syndrome associated with limbic system dysfunction. *J. Nerv. Ment. Dis.,* 164:56-63, 1977.

Vandereycken, W., & Meermann, R. *Anorexia Nervosa: A Clinician's Guide to Treatment.* Berlin, New York: Walter DeGruyter, 1984.

Walsh, B. T., Stewart, J., & Wright, L. Treatment of bulimia with monoamine oxidase inhibitors. *Am. J. Psychiatry,* 139:1629-1630, 1982.

Wegner, J. R., & Struve, F. A. Incidence of the 14 and 6-per-second positive spike pattern in an adult clinical population: An empirical note. *J. Nerv. Ment. Dis.,* 164:340-345, 1977.

Weiss, T., & Levitz, L. Piphenylhydantoin treatment of bulimia. (Letter) *Am. J. Psychiatry,* 133:1093, 1976.

Wermuth, B. M., Davis, K. L., Hollister, L. E., & Stunkard, A. J. Phenytoin treatment of the binge eating syndrome. *Am. J. Psychiatry,* 134:1249-1253, 1977.

White, J. H., & Schnaultz, N. L. Successful treatment of anorexia nervosa with imipramine. *Dis. Nerv. System,* 38:567-568, 1977.

Whittier, J. R. (Letter) Asphyxiation, bulimia and insulin levels in Huntington's Disease. *JAMA,* 235(14):1423, 1976.

Wilkus, R. J., & Chiles, J. A. Electrophysiological changes during episodes of the Klein-Levin Syndrome. *J. Neurol. Neurosurg. Psychiatry,* 38:1225-1231, 1975.

Winokur, A., March, V., & Mendels, J. Primary affective disorder in relatives of patients with anorexia nervosa. *Am. J. Psychiatry,* 137:697-698, 1980.

7

Serotonin in Eating Disorders: Theory and Therapy

David S. Goldbloom

Biological therapy of eating disorders is in its infancy, and speculations about its future are presumptuous. Nevertheless, the trend in clinical psychopharmacology is to increase the specificity of drug treatments to match the growing basic scientific understanding of the disorders. The advance of antipsychotic drugs from the early phenothiazines to the more recent diphenylbutylpiperidines reflects this process. In the arena of eating disorders, tricyclic antidepressants (Herzog & Brotman, Chapter 2, this volume), monoamine oxidase inhibitors (Kennedy & Walsh, Chapter 1, this volume), and anticonvulsants (Kaplan, Chapter 6, this volume) have been the focus of therapy over the last few years. These treatments have outstripped our understanding of the biological dysfunctions in eating disorders, and these drugs have multiple effects on brain

---

The author gratefully acknowledges the support of a Centennial Fellowship from the Medical Research Council of Canada during the preparation of this chapter. He also thanks Dr. Donald Coscina and Dr. Paul Garfinkel for their comments on earlier versions of portions of this chapter and Ms. Margaret Fardoe for the technical preparation of the manuscript.

neurotransmitters and receptors. Among these effects is enhancement of central serotoninergic transmission.

The brain neurotransmitter serotonin (5HT) has been the subject of intense scrutiny in biological psychiatry; serotoninergic dysfunction has been implicated in disorders of mood, suicidality, alcoholism, and aggression. The breadth of this research has been reviewed elsewhere (Van Praag, 1984). At the physiological level, research on 5HT has included investigation of its role in the control of appetite. This line of inquiry is only a decade old; a major text on 5HT and behavior published in 1973 did not include any mention of feeding (Barchas & Usdin, 1973). In order to hypothesize about new therapies involving 5HT in eating disorders, it is necessary to review first the evidence at a basic science level.

SEROTONIN AND FEEDING

Twenty-five years ago, Anand and Brobeck first proposed a neuroanatomical model for the hypothalamic control of food intake in rats, featuring a feeding center in the lateral hypothalamus and a satiety center in the ventromedial area (Anand & Brobeck, 1951). The evolution of understanding of brain control of eating behavior since that time reflects a shift to more dynamic and complex models of the central nervous system involving neurotransmitters and cybernetics.

A variety of monoamines, peptides, and amino acids have been shown to act as central neuropharmacological modulators of feeding behavior in animals (Blundell, 1984a; Morley & Levine, 1985). This is only logical; anything as basic to an organism's survival as regulating its energy balance should have multiple inputs and controls. At first glance, this may suggest that consideration of any single component fails to reflect systems interaction and interdependence; however, both animal and human data point to specific roles for neuromodulatory substances that may have both pathogenic and therapeutic roles in eating disorders.

Hunger and satiety in humans represent an admixture of physiological, psychological, and environmental inputs that are difficult to tease apart and measure; in laboratory animals, hunger and satiety are defined operationally via feeding behaviors. The hypothalamic model of feeding control integration in rats has survived advances in neuropharmacology in terms of the lateral area integrating "start feeding" inputs and the medial area integrating "stop feeding" inputs (Grossman, 1984; Hoebel, 1984).

In the medial hypothalamus, the neurotransmitter 5HT facilitates the "stop feeding" process in rats under experimental conditions (Blundell, 1984b). Intraventricular injections of 5HT and its precursors in rats depress feeding even in food-deprived rats. Similar results have been obtained with intraperitoneal injections of the 5HT precursors 5-hydroxytryptophan (5-HTP) and tryptophan (TRP) (Blundell, 1977). Further, the use of dietary TRP as a means to increase central 5HT synthesis influences eating behavior both in animals (Li & Anderson, 1983) and in humans (Hrboticky, Leiter, & Anderson, 1985). Other drugs whose influence is to increase presynaptic release of 5HT—such as fenfluramine—or to block its presynaptic reuptake—such as fluoxetine—decrease food intake and hasten the termination of feeding in food-deprived rats (Blundell, Latham, & Lesham, 1976; Goudie, Thornton, & Wheeler, 1976). Suppression of eating in humans has also been demonstrated with fenfluramine in obesity (Stunkard, Rickels, & Hessbacher, 1973) and in bulimia nervosa (Robinson, Checkley, & Russell, 1985). Fluoxetine has recently been shown to produce weight loss in nondepressed obese subjects (Ferguson, 1985). Of particular interest, fluoxetine has been reported specifically to elevate hypothalamic levels of 5HT (Fuller, Perry, & Molloy, 1974). Thus, experimental stimulation of serotoninergic pathways is associated with a suppression of food intake. In a recent review, Blundell indicated that the converse of this effect, the stimulation of food intake by suppression of serotoninergic pathways, is a demonstrable but much weaker phenomenon (Blundell, 1984b). This latter point has important implications for the pharmacological treatment of the restricting form of anorexia nervosa, and is discussed later in this chapter.

Although these studies suggest that 5HT is involved in satiety or in the general termination of feeding behavior, there is evidence for a more precise role for 5HT in the regulation of macronutrient intake composition. The ability of both fenfluramine and fluoxetine, but not amphetamine, to suppress selectively carbohydrate but not protein consumption in rats has been interpreted as serotoninergic control over carbohydrate (CHO) intake (Wurtman & Wurtman, 1977). Further, to complete the feedback loop, central serotoninergic activity is itself subject to dietary manipulation in some (Li & Anderson, 1982; Anderson & Johnston, 1983) but not all (Trulson, 1985) species. Dietary influence on 5HT metabolism has the following sequence (Wurtman & Wurtman, 1984b): CHO intake stimulates insulin secretion; insulin drives the large neutral amino acids (LNAAs) such as leucine, isoleucine, valine, tyrosine, and phenylalanine out of plasma and into tissue; however, TRP, an amino acid and 5HT precursor, remains in plasma, and thus its ratio to the other LNAAs is increased. A single competitive transport mechanism of LNAAs across the blood-brain barrier elevates brain TRP levels when the TRP/LNAA ratio increases. The enzyme TRP hydroxylase, which catalyzes the first step in the conversion of TRP to 5HT, is normally unsaturated with substrate. Thus, an increased availability of brain TRP leads to an increase in brain 5HT synthesis.

Dietary manipulation of brain 5HT through the above sequence has shown that, in rats, CHO loading, with a presumptive increase in brain 5HT, influences the rats to choose away from CHO when presented with food. Similarly, CHO-deficient diets, with a presumptive decrease in brain 5HT, direct rats to increase relative CHO consumption subsequently (Li & Anderson, 1984; Wurtman, Moses, & Wurtman, 1982). Similar effects have been observed in humans of normal weight; oral TRP (Hrboticky, Leiter, & Anderson, 1985) and fenfluramine (Wurtman & Wurtman, 1984a) selectively reduced CHO intake.

However, the relationship between dietary intake, 5HT activity, and feeding behavior in patients with anorexia nervosa and bulimia nervosa remains largely unexplored. Limits to this exploration in human subjects include the difficulty of manipulating or measuring hypothalamic 5HT without interference from other 5HT sources in the brain and in the periphery.

SEROTONIN AND EATING DISORDERS

Monoamine activity in anorexia nervosa and bulimia nervosa has received increasing attention in the last decade. Stimuli for this line of investigation include the known effects of the monoamines on the control of food intake and the clinical association between eating disorders and affective disorders.

At the outset, the limitations of current techniques to assess central monoamine function must be stressed. Especially important is the concern about whether assessments based on blood, urine, or cerebrospinal fluid (CSF) measures provide an accurate estimate of CNS monoamine activity. Furthermore, the effect of weight loss per se on monoamine metabolism limits interpretation of data in both the anorexic and bulimic patients who remain below their premorbid or ideal body weight. For example, urinary catecholamine metabolite excretion is related to percentage of body fat in normal-weight women (Johnston, Warsh, & Anderson, 1983) and in women with anorexia nervosa (Johnston, Leiter, Burrow, Garfinkel, et al., 1984).

With regard to 5HT metabolism, one of the earliest studies in anorexia nervosa examined TRP levels (Coppen, Gupta, & Eccleston, et al., 1976). A deficit in plasma TRP levels in underweight anorexics prior to therapeutic refeeding was observed relative to controls; after weight gain, total plasma TRP increased to control values, whereas nonprotein-bound TRP remained significantly low. Unfortunately, this study failed to provide more meaningful detail about the relationship of TRP to 5HT such as the TRP/LNAA ratio or levels of 5HT metabolites.

More recently, our group conducted a controlled study of six female anorexics. They showed both a reduced fasting plasma TRP and a reduced TRP/LNAA ratio, suggesting decreased TRP availability for central 5HT synthesis and ultimately diminished central serotoninergic activity (Johnston et al., 1984). This would be at variance with a theoretical rationale for the use of cyproheptadine, an antiserotoninergic drug, in anorexia nervosa (see below).

Similarly, a case report of markedly decreased CSF levels of 5-hydroxyindolacetic acid (5-HIAA), a 5HT metabolite, in two emaciated anorexics suggests central 5HT dysregulation of unknown etiology (Gillberg, 1983). Decreased urinary excretion of 5HT metabolites has also been reported in underweight patients with anorexia nervosa (Riederen, Toifl, & Kruzik, 1982).

Studies of 5HT metabolites in CSF have provided interesting if conflicting results. One controlled study of 33 underweight females with anorexia nervosa failed to show any differences in CSF 5-HIAA (Gerner, Cohen, & Fairbanks, 1984). This study assessed 5-HIAA at one point in time, and probenicid was not used to counter the efflux of 5-HIAA out of the CSF. Another study compared eight underweight anorexics with eight recently weight-recovered anorexics, eight long-term weight-recovered anorexics, and eight normal controls (Kaye, Ebert, Raleigh, & Lake, 1984a). Long-term weight-recovered anorexics had significantly higher CSF 5-HIAA levels than underweight anorexics, and among almost all of the underweight anorexics, weight gain was associated with an increase in 5-HIAA. The low 5-HIAA values in the underweight group could not be explained on the basis of deficient amino acid precursors.

Subsequent analysis of data from the same patients using probenicid blockade of 5-HIAA efflux from CSF revealed significant differences between the restricting and bulimic anorexics (Kaye, Ebert, Gwirtsman, & Weiss, 1984b). Weight-recovered bulimic patients had lower 5-HIAA levels than weight-recovered restricting anorexics or controls.

The implications of a relative hyposerotoninergic state in the bulimic subgroup of patients even after weight recovery are theoretical, clinical, and therapeutic. Especially important may be the role of 5HT in producing a self-perpetuating bulimia-restriction state leading to chronicity (Garfinkel & Kaplan, 1985). Animal studies of feeding demonstrate, as noted previously, that reduction of brain 5HT leads to increased CHO intake. Bulimic patients often binge on CHO-rich foods, and the failure for brain 5HT to reach normal levels with weight recovery may contribute to the perpetuation of bingeing behavior in normal-weight bulimics.

Interestingly, a similar hyposerotoninergic state has been proposed to explain the perpetuation of alcoholic behavior (Goodwin, 1985). Alcohol appears to increase 5HT activity as measured peripherally by platelet 5HT uptake during acute intoxication and then reduce 5HT to subnormal levels. It is argued that this biphasic effect on 5HT sets up a self-perpetuating mechanism for alcohol consumption. In rats, this biphasic effect of alcohol on 5HT parameters has been demonstrated (Badawy & Evans, 1976). Similarly, a study of CSF 5-HIAA in humans showed significantly lower 5-HIAA levels in alcoholics who had been abstinent for four weeks as compared with nonalcoholic personality-disordered controls (Ballenger, Goodwin, Major, & Brown, 1979). In the immediate postintoxication state, 5-HIAA was not significantly different between patients and controls. Given the ability of alcohol in rats to increase brain 5HT, this suggests a chronic hyposerotoninergic state in humans, which alcoholics self-medicate with alcohol.

Similarities between alcoholism and eating disorders may exist not only at a level of serotoninergic aberrations but also at a psychological level. Anorexia nervosa has been conceptualized as an addiction to starvation (Szmukler & Tantam, 1984) and bulimia nervosa may be seen as an irresistible impulse toward food abuse. Parallels between alcohol intoxication and starvation abound, including cognitive preoccupation, tolerance, and withdrawal symptoms. A further link between alcoholism and eating disorders is the high incidence of substance abuse among bulimic patients (Garfinkel, Moldofsky, & Garner, 1980) and the increased incidence of alcoholism in their families (Strober, Salkin, Burroughs, & Morrell, 1982). Presumably an interplay of genetic and environmental factors accounts for this overlap. Nevertheless, it is relevant to this discussion that recent therapeutic trials in alcoholism have included serotoninergic drugs such as zimelidine (Naranjo, Sellers, Wu, & Lawrin, 1985), and that at an animal level 5HT may inhibit preference for alcohol (Hytell & Larsen, 1985).

CYPROHEPTADINE

The entry of cyproheptadine into the arena of psychopharmacology reflects a serendipity paralleled by the examples of iproniazid and chlorpromazine. Cyproheptadine came to clinical attention in 1959 as a potential therapeutic agent in allergic asthma and hay fever (Lavenstein, 1962). In the laboratory, its capacity for antagonism of 5HT and histamine was established (Stone, Wenger, Ludden, Stavorski, & Ross, 1961) at a time when little was known of the relevance of 5HT to psychiatry in general and appetite in particular.

The first recognition of an association between cyproheptadine, appetite, and weight gain emerged from a double-blind comparison with the antihistamine chlorpheniramine in children with bronchial asthma (Lavenstein, 1962). Although both drugs provided equivalent asthma relief, patients receiving cyproheptadine showed over twice the mean weight gain as patients on chlorpheniramine. In the context of a crossover design, this unanticipated effect of cyproheptadine rapidly disappeared when patients were switched to chlorpheniramine. Qualitative and informal assessment of appetite revealed an increase with cyproheptadine. The authors acknowledged the failure of dog and rat studies of cyproheptadine to reproduce these effects on appetite and weight in a more carefully designed and controlled trial and were appropriately unable to explain the mechanism by which cyproheptadine appeared to increase appetite. Indeed, these limitations foreshadowed developments in both basic scientific and clinical research. A final irony is the citation in this 1962 paper of the work on obesity by Hilde Bruch, whose later writings on anorexia nervosa were paralleled by later applications of cyproheptadine to the treatment of that disorder.

Two more studies in the 1960s laid the foundation for the trials of cyproheptadine in eating disorders in the 1970s. Another sample of underweight, chronically hospitalized, severely asthmatic children were treated with either placebo or 16 mg per day of cyproheptadine for 15 weeks with specific attention to parameters of growth and appetite. Without any impact on asthmatic status, cyproheptadine again showed a significant increase in weight in this population and an unquantified increase in appetite. Again, the author acknowledged the failure of cyproheptadine to induce weight gain in a variety of laboratory animals and, based on unpublished data, in adults (Bergen, 1964). The majority of subjects in this study were in the preadolescent phase of rapid growth, and even the placebo group showed significant weight gain.

In another study, 20 adult outpatients who were, on average, 13 pounds below actuarially defined ideal body weight received either placebo or 12 mg per day of cyproheptadine for 56 days (Noble, 1969). The patients were determined to be in satisfactory health, and neither the origins of their underweight nor their motivation for seeking treatment were stated; under the circumstances of the study, however, there must have been considerable motivation on the part of the subjects to gain weight. Indeed, a mean increase in appetite and weight gain was seen in both the placebo and cyproheptadine groups, with a mean gain of 1.3 kg in the former and 3.8 kg in the latter group over 56 days. Drowsiness as a side effect occurred in 50% of patients on cyproheptadine, but in no patients on placebo. Thus, maintenance of double-blind conditions was likely limited among these patients desiring to gain weight. Further, drowsiness as a harness on activity may have had some impact on caloric expenditure and weight.

These three studies formed the basis for subsequent clinical investigation and use of cyproheptadine in stimulation of appetite and promotion of weight gain. Two of these studies involved children with significant physical illnesses during periods of natural growth, and one studied a population that may have had high hopes of weight gain. No theory or animal model explained the clinical results. A fourth study of the effects of 12 mg per day of cyproheptadine differed from the above three studies in that the population examined featured 12 healthy adults (Stiel, Liddle, & Lacy, 1970). By controlling dietary intake in a subgroup of three subjects, the authors reported a consistent effect of drowsiness with cyproheptadine "sufficient to reduce normal activity" that could have accounted for the slight weight increase seen on cyproheptadine with a constant diet.

Use of cyproheptadine in anorexia nervosa began with a 1970 case report (Benady, 1970). A 14-year-old girl, with a two-year history of anorexia nervosa refractory to psychotherapy, high-dose antipsychotic medication, and hospitalization, was treated with cyproheptadine 12 mg per day in addition to psychotherapy. Over 10 months she gained 30 pounds, and the cyproheptadine was discontinued. She had maintained her weight gain at six-month follow-up. The usual scientific limitations to a single case report apply here, especially in terms of two simultaneous treatments and the lack of a placebo crossover design. Indeed, the ability of this patient to sustain weight gain off cyproheptadine was contrary to the previous studies in which patients lost weight upon discontinuation of the medication. Nevertheless, in the context of refractoriness of some anorexic patients to standard intervention, the appeal of such a case report is evident.

Meanwhile, improved scientific studies of cyproheptadine in other populations began to consider the role of 5HT in feeding. A study of 16 "thin but otherwise normal university students who had all expressed a desire to gain weight" (Silverstone & Schuyler, 1975) tested 12 mg per day of cyproheptadine against placebo in a double-blind crossover design. Almost half the subjects failed to complete the eight-week study, with severe cyproheptadine-induced drowsiness as the most common reason; eight of the nine subjects who completed the study reported drowsiness on cyproheptadine. Weight and hunger increased on cyproheptadine and the authors pondered whether this reflected the blockade of an inhibitory serotoninergic control on feeding.

The first double-blind trial of cyproheptadine in anorexia nervosa appeared in 1977 (Vigersky & Loriaux, 1977). This eight-week trial tested 12 mg per day of cyproheptadine versus placebo in 24 patients meeting research diagnostic criteria for anorexia nervosa. No side effects of cyproheptadine were reported in this outpatient trial. Despite randomization, certain characteristics of the cyproheptadine group distinguished it from the placebo group: it was significantly older, longer in duration of illness, and more prone to drug abuse in promotion of weight loss. Thirty-one percent of patients on cyproheptadine and 18% on placebo gained weight; the differences between the two treatments were not statistically significant in terms of numbers of reponders or amount of weight gain. The authors highlighted the importance of recognizing limits in comparing their population to others studied with cyproheptadine—that anorexia nervosa is unique in its feature of "the relentless pursuit of thinness." Nevertheless, limitations to this study included the presence of bulimic behaviors interfering with absorption and an outpatient trial limiting compliance.

Since then, Halmi and colleagues have been the chief proponents of further study of cyproheptadine in anorexia nervosa. Their first report (Goldberg, Halmi, & Eckert, 1979) showed a significant effect of cyproheptadine on weight gain in subgroups of anorexia nervosa, such as among those with a history of two or more birth delivery complications. The reason for such a difference among a small subgroup of six patients is unclear. Other responding subgroups to cyproheptadine in doses of up to 32 mg per day included those with severe weight loss and those with a history of prior outpatient treatment failure. That the authors encountered no side effects, such as drowsiness, at high doses is surprising in view of previous experiences with cyproheptadine. Neither the length of treatment nor the period of follow-up was described in this first report and effects of cyproheptadine on measures other than weight gain were not included. Subsequently, however, this group reported on an expanded sample of 105 anorexic patients (Goldberg, Eckert, Halmi, et al., 1980). Here a global effect of cyproheptadine on characteristic attitudinal and behavioral features of anorexia nervosa was described. It is unstated whether, in multivariate analysis, these psychologically oriented changes were independent of weight gain. It is well known that many of the cognitive preoccupations and personality characteristics of anorexia nervosa are accentuated by weight loss (Garfinkel & Garner, 1982). It is unclear whether these same psychological changes are seen in noncyproheptadine-mediated recovery from anorexia nervosa.

These same investigators subsequently conducted an inpatient trial of cyproheptadine versus amitriptyline versus placebo in anorexia nervosa (Halmi, Eckert, & Falk, 1982, 1983). A total of 57 subjects were treated with 32 mg of cyproheptadine per day, 160 mg per day of amitriptyline, or placebo. Although the mean percent of target weight increased in the cyproheptadine group from 81% to 98%, it is noticeable that the placebo group demonstrated a mean increase from 75% to 89%. Indeed, the effect of amitriptyline or cyproheptadine versus placebo was significant but not highly so.

All three groups showed a mean weight increase in the seven days between admission and starting the drug trial, and this was greatest in the cyproheptadine group, which suggests intergroup differences may have influenced the drug outcome. Further, depression ratings showed a significant effect for cyproheptadine over amitriptyline or placebo. Given a maximum dose of 160 mg per day of amitriptyline, it is possible that some patients received subtherapeutic doses; plasma levels were not reported. In a recent related publication, these authors have demonstrated quantitatively that cyproheptadine diminished motor activity in the first two weeks of inpatient treatment of women with anorexia nervosa (Falk, Halmi, & Tryon, 1985).

The most recent published analysis of the data from this inpatient trial has provided new perspectives on cyproheptadine (Halmi, Eckert, LaDu, & Cohen, 1986). By means of a newly generated measure of treatment efficiency, cyproheptadine was shown to produce a significantly poorer outcome among anorexics of the bulimic subtype; the authors cautioned against the use of cyproheptadine in such patients. Further, in contrast to these authors' 1979 report, no effect of cyproheptadine on symptoms and attitudes in anorexia nervosa was seen. Both amitriptyline and cyproheptadine provided only modest advantages over placebo for the group as a whole in terms of number of patients achieving target weight, number of days to target weight, and average rate of weight gain. Changes in depression ratings were intimately linked with weight gain.

Significant limitations remain to the role of cyproheptadine in the treatment of anorexia nervosa. At a clinical level, these patients do not suffer from true loss of appetite until late in the course of their illness (Garfinkel & Garner, 1982); indeed, they are cognitively preoccupied by food. Much as obesity is a syndrome rather than a disease, the emaciation seen in anorexia nervosa differs markedly from that seen in the other disorders in which cyproheptadine has been shown to increase weight.

At a research level, problems with particular studies have already been indicated. The results of Halmi and colleagues have not been replicated by other groups in the published literature and stand in contrast to the findings of Vigersky and Loriaux. At a basic science level, the effects of cyproheptadine have been somewhat contradictory. As described previously, early investigators failed to demonstrate an appetite-stimulating effect in several animal species. Highly variable, insignificant, and even anorexigenic effects have been observed in rats (Blavet, DeFeudis, & Clostre, 1982; Chakrabarty, Bhatnagar, & Chakrabarty, 1974). Finally, at a theoretical level, a rationale for the use of cyproheptadine is its putative ability to block serotoninergically mediated inhibition of feeding. There is no evidence of "serotoninergic overdrive" in anorexia nervosa at this time. However, cyproheptadine does increase electrical activity in the lateral hypothalamus—the "feeding center"—in cats (Chakrabarty, Pillai, Anand, & Singh, 1967); in rats it both activates lateral hypothalamic neurons and inhibits neurons in the ventromedial hypothalamus—the satiety center (Oomura, Ono, Sugimori, & Nakamura, 1973).

Cyproheptadine may have a future role in pharmacotherapy of

eating disorders and other psychiatric disorders; it has been of use at an anecdotal level in the treatment of tricyclic and MAOI—antidepressant-induced anorgasmia (Sovner, 1984; DeCastro, 1985) and in the treatment of depression (Bansal & Brown, 1983). Additional confirmation of the benefit of cyproheptadine in the treatment of the particular thinness that is anorexia nervosa is needed before it can be endorsed for clinical use. Future studies should include measures of serotoninergic activity and assess whether this is the mode of action of cyproheptadine.

TRYPTOPHAN

Given a hypothesis of serotoninergic modulation of satiety, tryptophan (TRP) appears a "natural" means of increasing 5HT synthesis and activity in the brain. Over two decades of psychiatric research with TRP have focused on its potential in the treatment of affective disorders with equivocal or modestly positive outcome (Byerley & Risch, 1985; Young, 1984).

The extensive animal literature of TRP is not reviewed here. The use of TRP and its metabolite, 5-hydroxytryptophan (5-HTP), as 5HT precursors have generated much animal data supporting the role of 5HT in feeding. More recently, human studies have focused on the effects of TRP on food choice and intake. A series of investigations of individuals with self-reported CHO craving have tested the impact of TRP on feeding behavior (Wurtman & Wurtman, 1984). Within this population, 2 grams of TRP an hour prior to a snack did not significantly reduce CHO intake despite a trend in that direction (Wurtman & Wurtman, 1984a). A second study included eight subjects treated with 800 mg of TRP three times a day and again showed a reduction in CHO snack number in three subjects, whereas four showed no change and one significantly increased CHO snack intake (Wurtman et al., 1981).

More pronounced effects were seen with fenfluramine in these studies. Despite their propensity to snack preferentially on CHO, none of these subjects engaged in clinical bulimic behaviors. The limited response to TRP in some subjects is evocative of outcome in studies of TRP in the treatment of affective disorders. Further, the dose of TRP used is low relative to doses used in humans to demonstrate the effect of oral TRP on central 5HT (Eccleston, Ashcroft, Crawford, et al., 1970) and to treat bipolar disorder (Chouinard, Young, & Annable, 1985).

More precise measurement of the effect of TRP on short-term energy and macronutrient consumption lends further support for 5HT in the control of feeding (Hrboticky, Leiter, & Anderson, 1985). Lean, healthy males were given a standardized breakfast after an overnight fast. One hour prior to a luncheon buffet, they received 2 grams of TRP or placebo on each of four test days. A significant reduction in total energy intake at lunch occurred with doses of 2 and 3 grams of TRP, but did not occur at 1-gram doses. Similarly, a reduction in CHO food choices relative to protein choices occurred only with doses of 2 and 3 grams. Doses of 3 grams of TRP significantly reduced the urge to eat as measured on a visual analogue scale. Thus, whereas doses of 2 grams or more of TRP were needed to demonstrate an acute effect, at these doses significantly decreased alertness also occurred.

Although there is good reason to believe that the anorexic effect of TRP is distinct from its psychotropic effect, these effects—as well as the contribution of peripheral effects of TRP—are difficult to tease apart in human studies. Apart from the extensive work of Wurtman and colleagues in the treatment of obese CHO-cravers, there has been only one reported trial of TRP in eating disorders. TRP in doses of 1 gram three times per day was not significantly different from placebo among 13 patients with bulimia nervosa (Krahn & Mitchell, 1985). However, multiple design flaws limit the significance of this study. It was conducted in outpatients with no measures of compliance or absorption-significant issues in an impulsive and purging population. Relative to other studies of TRP, the dose employed may well have been subtherapeutic in terms of modulation of satiety. However, nausea and sedation may prove to be limiting factors at higher doses.

Current evidence is inadequate to indicate a therapeutic role for TRP in the clinical treatment of anorexia nervosa or bulimia nervosa. However, theoretical understanding of satiety and its disorders justifies further research. Future trials of TRP in bulimia nervosa should include peripheral indices of central 5HT metabolism, TRP/LNAA ratios, measures of hunger and satiety, and evaluation of macronutrient selection. Such detailed assessment is necessary to establish a clinical role for this relatively nontoxic therapeutic agent.

FENFLURAMINE

Dextro-fenfluramine enhances release of 5HT from presynaptic terminals and inhibits reuptake. Its potential as an anorexic agent has been studied for over a decade and it is currently among the standard drugs used in the pharmacological treatment of obesity (Galloway, Farquhar, & Munro, 1984). Studies of fenfluramine relevant to obesity are not reviewed here.

At a basic science level, more precise definition of the anorexigenic effect of fenfluramine is of relevance to eating disorders. Unlike the anorexic agent amphetamine, fenfluramine does not delay the onset of feeding in rats; rather, it reduces meal size and hastens the termination of feeding (Blundell, Latham, & Lesham, 1976). This effect is consistent with a serotoninergic mediation of satiety and may be significant in the treatment of bingeing behavior. More recent confirmation of the effects of norfenfluramine, a fenfluramine metabolite, in rats includes decreases in meal size, rate of consumption, and carbohydrate intake, while maintaining protein intake and normal latency to meal onset (Leibowitz, 1985).

A recent study of the acute effects of fenfluramine on binge behavior in patients with bulimia nervosa yielded interesting if preliminary results (Robinson, Checkley, & Russell, 1985). Fifteen bulimic females were given either a single dose of fenfluramine 60 mg or placebo after an overnight fast. Two hours after drug administration, patients were left alone with a liberal supply of foods on which they were likely to binge. Fenfluramine significantly reduced food intake compared to placebo. Food intake on placebo was significantly greater than for nonbulimic control patients given placebo in the same test paradigm. None of the postfenfluramine meals was rated by bulimics as a binge, whereas six of 15 postplacebo meals were rated as near or definite binges, and a further three subjects binged within a few hours after the test. Macronutrient selection was not measured precisely. Visual analogue scales demonstrated a postprandial decrease in the urge to eat on fenfluramine that was significantly greater than that seen after placebo. The major side effect of fenfluramine was drowsiness.

Limitations to this study include a laboratory setting for bingeing behavior that cannot simulate completely a binge environment and the brevity of the study period; side effects may have helped both in reducing food intake and in distinguishing between active drug and placebo. Further, the question of a peripheral effect of fenfluramine mediating its reduction in caloric intake was not addressed. Nevertheless, the results are consistent with a serotoninergic satiety model and may indicate a therapeutic role in bulimia nervosa; an extended outpatient trial of fenfluramine is in progress (Robinson, personal communication).

An investigation directed to more precise quantification of macronutrient intake examined the effect of fenfluramine in 20 obese patients who claimed to crave CHO as an intermeal snack (Wurtman, Wurtman, Mark, et al., 1985). Fenfluramine significantly reduced total caloric intake through a reduction in CHO intake both at meals and during snacks; this effect was more pronounced at snacks than at meals. This corroborates animal data and distinguishes the anorexic effect of fenfluramine from the more global anorexia of amphetamine. Whether such effects can be replicated in a bulimic population remains to be seen. Currently, the use of fenfluramine in this particular population must be regarded as experimental.

FLUOXETINE

Fluoxetine is an investigational drug that has been undergoing extensive clinical trials, chiefly in affective disorders, in recent years. It is a potent and highly selective inhibitor of 5HT uptake into brain synapses, a feature in common with some traditional antidepressants (Wong, Bymaster, Horng, & Molloy, 1975). Its putative mode of action is via 5HT uptake blockade leading to increased 5HT availability for neurotransmission, without significant direct effect on catecholamine uptake or postsynaptic receptor sensitivity (Stark, Fuller, & Wong, 1985).

Clinical trials of fluoxetine have shown it to be an antidepressant with comparable therapeutic effect to amitriptyline (Chouinard, 1985), although significant weight gain was more prominent in the amitriptyline patients. In a comparative trial with imipramine, therapeutic effect was again equivalent to that seen with a traditional antidepressant, but the fluoxetine responders were characterized by features of chronic, early onset, and atypical depression—important in terms of the mood disorders encountered in eating-disordered patients (Reimherr, Wood, & Byerley, 1984).

At a preclinical level, investigation of the ability of fluoxetine to modulate feeding behavior has yielded interesting results. The knowledge that fluoxetine selectively elevates hypothalamic 5HT (Fuller, Perry, & Molloy, 1974) prompted the testing of its ability to promote satiety. A transient but potent anorexic effect has been demonstrated in rats (Goudie, Thornton, & Wheeler, 1976); paralleling the evolution of understanding of the role of 5HT in eating, fluoxetine has been shown to reduce total caloric intake in rats while sparing protein consumption (Wurtman & Wurtman, 1977). Further, in contrast to fenfluramine tested in the same paradigm, tolerance to the anorexic effect of fluoxetine in rats is absent (Rowland, Antelman, & Kocan, 1982). Suppression of appetite and reduction of body weight occurs in both normal and obese mice treated with fluoxetine (Wong & Yen, 1985).

Clinical studies of fluoxetine in patients with eating disorders are limited. One study of 150 nonbulimic obese outpatients tested fluoxetine against benzamphetamine or placebo (Ferguson, 1986). None of the subjects was depressed on psychometric evaluation. Fluoxetine proved an effective anorexic agent for this significantly obese (average weight 203 lb), largely female population. Patients with marked self-reported CHO-craving on a visual analogue scale lost the most weight, whereas similarly craving patients on placebo lost the least weight. However, an effect similar to that of fluoxetine was seen with benzamphetamine as well, suggesting a nonspecific effect. An informal aspect of the study asked subjects how they felt the drug had influenced their eating patterns. Many fluoxetine subjects reported earlier onset of satiety associated with normal meals and earlier termination of feeding. This is of interest in the context of bingeing behavior where the normal satiety signals are not operative.

An open-label, uncontrolled study of fluoxetine in 10 patients with clinically significant bulimia and varying degrees of depressive symptomatology has yielded tantalizing results which are tempered by the limits of such a study design (Freeman, 1985). A dramatic reduction in bingeing and purging occurred in nine out of 10 subjects within a few weeks on fluoxetine. The drug was prescribed at antidepressant dosages, and this preliminary investigation does not adequately distinguish an antibulimic effect from an antidepressant effect.

A multicenter, double-blind, placebo-controlled investigation of fluoxetine in bulimia nervosa is underway, examining the largest cohort of bulimic subjects ever studied with a single therapeutic agent in one protocol. Measures will be used to attempt to delineate more precisely an antibulimic effect. Nevertheless, clinicians recognize dysphoric mood states in the context of bulimia nervosa, and it will likely be impossible to control completely for an antidepressant effect. Should fluoxetine prove efficacious, it will be studied in comparison to the more nonspecific tricyclic antidepressants in the treatment of bulimia nervosa.

CONCLUSION

It is unlikely that there will be a silver bullet for the treatment of any particular eating disorder. Nevertheless, just as the sensitivity of microorganisms to a variety of different antibiotics may be determined, a subset of eating-disordered patients may be responsive to specific agents. Greater understanding of the biological aberrancies in some of these patients may be paralleled by the development of newer generations of highly specific psychotropic drugs. 5HT is only one model that has pathogenic and therapeutic potential; at a clinical level, this and other biological models must be accommodated within the psychological and cultural contexts of eating disorders.

REFERENCES

Anand, B. K., & Brobeck, J. R. Hypothalamic control of food intake in rats and cats. *Yale J. Biol. Med.,* 24:123–140, 1951.

Anderson, G. H., & Johnston, J. L. Nutrient control of brain neurotransmitter synthesis and function. *Can. J. Physiol. Pharmacol.,* 61:271–281, 1983.

Badawy, A.A.B., & Evans, M. The role of free serum tryptophan in the biphasic effect of acute ethanol administration on the concentration of rat brain tryptophan, 5-hydroxytryptamine, and 5-hydroxyindole-3-acetic acid. *Biochem. J.,* 160:315–324, 1976.

Ballenger, J. C., Goodwin, F. K., Major, L. F., & Brown, G. L. Alcohol and central serotonin metabolism in man. *Arch. Gen. Psychiatry,* 36:224–227, 1979.

Bansal, S., & Brown, W. A. Cyproheptadine in depression. *Lancet,* ii:803, 1983.

Barchas, J., & Usdin, E. (Eds.). *Serotonin and Behavior.* New York: Academic Press, 1973.

Benady, D. R. Cyproheptadine hydrochloride (Periactin) and anorexia nervosa: A case report. *Br. J. Psychiatry,* 117:681–682, 1970.

Bergen, S. S. Appetite stimulating properties of cyproheptadine. *Am. J. Dis. Child.,* 108:270–273, 1964.

Blavet, N., DeFeudis, F. V., & Clostre, F. Inhibition of food intake in the rat by cyproheptadine. *Experientia,* 38:264–265, 1982.

Blundell, J. E. Is there a role for serotonin (5-hydroxytryptamine) in feeding? *Int. J. Obesity,* 1:15–42, 1977.

Blundell, J. E. Systems and interactions: An approach to the pharmacology of eating and hunger. In A. J. Stunkard & E. Stellar (Eds.), *Eating and Its Disorders.* New York: Raven Press, 1984a.

Blundell, J. E. Serotonin and appetite. *Neuropharmacol.,* 23:1537–1551, 1984b.

Blundell, J. E., Latham, C. J., & Lesham, M. B. Differences between the anorexic action of amphetamine and fenfluramine: Possible effects on hunger and satiety. *J. Pharm. Pharmacol.,* 28:471–477, 1976.

Byerley, W. F., & Risch, S. C. Depression and serotonin metabolism: Rationale for neurotransmitter precursor treatment. *J. Clin. Psychopharmacol,* 5:191–206, 1985.

Chakrabarty, A. S., Bhatnagar, O. P., & Chakrabarty, K. Feeding behaviour of cyproheptadine treated rats. *Indian J. Med. Res.,* 62:726–730, 1974.

Chakrabarty, A. S., Pillai, R. V., Anand, B. K., & Singh, B. Effect of cyproheptadine on the electrical activity of the hypothalamic feeding centres. *Brain Res.,* 6:561–569, 1967.

Chouinard, G. C. A double-blind controlled clinical trial of fluoxetine and amitriptyline in the treatment of outpatients with major depressive disorder. *J. Clin. Psychiatry,* 46:32–37, 1985.

Chouinard, G. C., Young, S. N., & Annable, L. A controlled clinical trial of L-tryptophan in acute mania. *Biol. Psychiat.,* 20:546–557, 1985.

Coppen, A. J., Gupta, R. K., Eccleston, E. G., Wood, K. M., Wakeling, A., & DaSousa, V.F.A. Plasma tryptophan in anorexia nervosa. *Lancet,* i:961, 1976.

DeCastro, R. M. Reversal of MAOI-induced anorgasmia with cyproheptadine. *Am. J. Psychiatry,* 142:783, 1985.

Eccleston, D., Ashcroft, G. W., Crawford, T.B.B., Stanton, J. B., Wood, D., & McTurk, P. H. Effect of tryptophan administration on 5-HIAA in cerebrospinal fluid in man. *J. Neurol. Neurosurg. Psychiat.*, 33:269–272, 1970.

Falk, J. R., Halmi, K. A., & Tryon, W. W. Activity measures in anorexia nervosa. *Arch. Gen. Psychiatry*, 42:811–814, 1985.

Ferguson, J.M. Fluoxetine-induced weight loss in overweight, nondepressed subjects. *Am. J. Psychiatry*, 143:1496, 1986.

Freeman, C. Unpublished data, 1985.

Fuller, R.W., Perry, K.W., & Molloy, B.B. Effect of an uptake inhibitor of serotonin metabolism in rat brain. *Life Sci.*, 15:1161–1171, 1974.

Galloway, S.M., Farquhar, D.L., & Munro, J.F. The current status of antiobesity drugs. *Postgrad. Med. J.*, 60:19–26, 1984.

Garfinkel, P.E., & Garner, D.M. *Anorexia Nervosa: A Multidimensional Perspective.* New York: Brunner/Mazel, 1982.

Garfinkel, P.E., & Kaplan, A.S. Starvation-based perpetuating mechanisms in anorexia nervosa and bulimia. *Int. J. Eating Disorders*, 4:651–665, 1985.

Garfinkel, P.E., Moldofsky, H., & Garner, D.M. The heterogeneity of anorexia nervosa: Bulimia as a distinct subgroup. *Arch. Gen. Psychiatry*, 37:1036–1040, 1980.

Gerner, R.H., Cohen, D.J., Fairbanks, L., Anderson, G.M., Young, J.G., Scheinin, M., Linnoila, M., Shaywitz, B.A., & Hare, T.A. CSF neurochemistry of women with anorexia nervosa and normal women. *Am. J. Psychiatry*, 141:1441–1444, 1984.

Gillberg, C. Low dopamine and serotonin levels in anorexia nervosa. *Am. J. Psychiatry*, 140:948–949, 1983.

Goldberg, S.C., Halmi, K.A., Eckert, E.D., Casper, R.C., & Davis, J.M. Cyproheptadine in anorexia nervosa. *Br. J. Psychiatry*, 134:67-170, 1979.

Goldberg, S.C., Eckert, E.D., Halmi, K.A., Davis, J.M., & Roper, M. Effects of cyproheptadine on symptoms and attitudes in anorexia nervosa. *Arch. Gen. Psychiatry*, 37:1083, 1980.

Goodwin, D.W. Alcoholism and genetics. *Arch. Gen. Psychiatry*, 42:171–174, 1985.

Goudie, A.J., Thornton, E.W., & Wheeler, T.J. Effects of Lilly 110 140, a specific inhibitor of 5-hydroxytryptamine uptake, on food intake and on 5-hydroxytryptophan-induced anorexia. Evidence for serotoninergic inhibition of feeding. *J. Pharm. Pharmacol.*, 28:318–320, 1976.

Grossman, S.P. Contemporary problems concerning our understanding of brain mechanisms that regulate food intake and body weight. In A. J. Stunkard & E. Stellar (Eds.), *Eating and Its Disorders*. New York: Raven Press, 1984.

Halmi, K.A., Eckert, E., & Falk, J.R. Cyproheptadine for anorexia nervosa. *Lancet*, i:1357–1358, 1982.

Halmi, K.A., Eckert, E., & Falk, J.R. Cyproheptadine, an antidepressant and weight-inducing drug for anorexia nervosa. *Psychopharmacol. Bull.*, 19:103–105, 1983.

Halmi, K.A., Eckert, E.D., LaDu, T.J., & Cohen, J. Anorexia nervosa: Treatment efficacy of cyproheptadine and amitriptyline. *Arch. Gen. Psychiatry*, 43:177–181, 1986.

Hoebel, B. G. Neurotransmitters in the control of feeding and its rewards: Monoamines, opiates, and brain-gut peptides. In A. J. Stunkard & E. Stellar (Eds.), *Eating and Its Disorders*. New York: Raven Press, 1984.

Hrboticky, N., Leiter, L.A., & Anderson, G.H. Effects of L-tryptophan on short-term food intake in lean men. *Nutr. Res.*, 5:595–607, 1985.

Hytell, J., & Larsen, J.J. Neuropharmacological mechanisms of serotonin re-uptake inhibitors. In C. A. Naranjo & E. M. Sellers (Eds.), *Research Advances in New Psychopharmacological Treatments for Alcoholism*. New York: Excerpta Medica, 1985.

Johnston, J.L., Leiter, L.A., Burrow, G.N., Garfinkel, P.E., & Anderson, G.H. Excretion of urinary catecholamine metabolites in anorexia nervosa: Effect of body composition and energy intake. *Am. J. Clin. Nutr.*, 40:1001–1006, 1984.

Johnston, J.F.L., Warsh, J.J., & Anderson, G.H. Obesity and precursor availability affect urinary catecholamine metabolite production in women. *Am J. Clin. Nutr.*, 38:356–368, 1983.

Kaye, W.H., Ebert, M.H., Raleigh, M., & Lake, C.R. Abnormalities in CNS monoamine metabolism in anorexia nervosa. *Arch. Gen. Psychiatry*, 41:350–355, 1984a.

Kaye, W.H., Ebert, M.H., Gwirtsman, H.E., & Weiss, S.R. Differences in brain serotonergic metabolism between nonbulimic and bulimic patients with anorexia nervosa. *Am. J. Psychiatry*, 141:1598–1601, 1984b.

Krahn, D., & Mitchell, J. Use of L-tryptophan in treating bulimia. *Am J. Psychiatry*, 142:1130, 1985.

Lavenstein, A.F., Dacaney, E.P., Lasagna, L., & Van Metre, T.E. Effect of cyproheptadine on asthmatic children. *JAMA,* 180:90–94, 1962.

Leibowitz, S.F. Brain neurotransmitters and appetite regulation. *Psychopharmacol. Bull.,* 21:412–418, 1985.

Li, E.T.S., & Anderson, G.H. Self-selected meal composition, circadian rhythms and meal responses in plasma and brain tryptophan and 5-hydroxytryptamine in rats. *J. Nutr.,* 112:2001–2010, 1982.

Li, E.T.S., & Anderson, G.H. Amino acids in the regulation of food intake. *Nutr. Abstr. Rev. Clin. Nutr.,* 53:169–181, 1983.

Li, E.T.S., & Anderson, G.H. 5-hydroxytryptamine: a modulator of food composition but not quantity? *Life Sci.,* 34:2453–2460, 1984.

Morley, J.E., & Levine, A.S. The pharmacology of eating behaviour. *Ann. Rev. Pharmacol. Toxicol.,* 25:127–146, 1985.

Naranjo, C.A., Sellers, E.M., Wu, P.H., & Lawrin, M.O. Moderation of ethanol drinking: Role of enhanced serotonergic transmission. In C.A. Naranjo & E.M. Sellers (Eds.), *Research Advances in New Psychopharmacological Treatments for Alcoholism.* New York: Excerpta Medica, 1985.

Noble, R.E. Effect of cyproheptadine on appetite and weight gain in adults. *JAMA,* 209:2054–2055, 1969.

Oomura, Y., Ono, T., Sugimori, M., & Nakamura, T. Effects of cyproheptadine on the feeding and satiety centres of the rat. *Pharmacol. Biochem. Behav.,* 1:449–459, 1973.

Reimherr, F.W., Wood, D.R., Byerley, B., Brainard, J., & Grosser, B.I. Characteristics of responders to fluoxetine. *Psychopharmacol. Bull.,* 20:70–72, 1984.

Riederen, P., Toifl, K., & Kruzik, P. Excretion of biogenic amine metabolites in anorexia nervosa. *Clin. Chim. Acta,* 123:27–32, 1982.

Robinson, P.H., Checkley, S.A., & Russell, G.F.M. Suppression of eating by fenfluramine in patients with bulimia nervosa. *Br. J. Psychiatry,* 146:169–176, 1985.

Rowland, N., Antelman, S.M., & Kocan, D. Differences among "serotoninergic" anorectics in a cross-tolerance paradigm: Do they all act on serotonin systems? *Eur. J. Pharmacol.,* 81:57–66, 1982.

Silverstone, J.T., & Schuyler, D. The effect of cyproheptadine on hunger, calorie intake, and body weight in man. *Psychopharmacologia,* 40:335–340, 1975.

Sovner, R. Treatment of tricyclic antidepressant-induced orgasmic inhibition with cyproheptadine. *J. Clin. Psychopharmacol.,* 4:169, 1984.

Stark, P., Fuller, R.W., & Wong, D.T. The pharmacologic profile of fluoxetine. *J. Clin. Psychiatry,* 46:7–13, 1985.

Stiel, J.N., Liddle, G.W., & Lacy, W.W. Studies of mechanism of cyproheptadine-induced weight gain in human subjects. *Metabolism,* 19:192–200, 1970.

Stone, C.A., Wenger, H.C., Ludden, C.T., Stavorski, J.M., & Ross, C.A. Antiserotonin-antihistaminic properties of cyproheptadine. *J. Pharmacol. Exp. Ther.,* 131:73–84, 1961.

Strober, M., Salkin, B., Burroughs, J., & Morrell, W. Validity of the bulimia-restrictor distinction in anorexia nervosa: Parental personality characteristics and family psychiatric morbidity. *J. Nerv. Ment. Dis.,* 170:345–351, 1982.

Stunkard, A.J., Rickels, J., & Hessbacher, P. Fenfluramine in the treatment of obesity. *Lancet,* ii:503–505, 1973.

Szmukler, G.I., & Tantam, D. Anorexia nervosa: Starvation dependence. *Br. J. Med. Psychol.,* 57:303–310, 1984.

Trulson, M.E. Dietary tryptophan does not alter the function of brain serotonin neurons. *Life Sci.,* 37:1067–1072, 1985.

Van Praag, H.M. Depression, suicide, and serotonin metabolism in the brain. In R.M. Post & J.C. Ballenger (Eds.), *Neurobiology of Mood Disorders.* Baltimore: Williams & Wilkins, 1984.

Vigersky, R.A., & Loriaux, D.L. The effect of cyproheptadine in anorexia nervosa: A double-blind trial. In R.A. Vigersky (Ed.), *Anorexia Nervosa.* New York: Raven Press, 1977.

Wong, D.T., Bymaster, F.P., Horng, J.S., & Molloy, B.B. A new selective inhibitor for uptake of serotonin into synaptosomes of rat brain: 3-(p-trifluoromethylphenoxy)-N-methyl-3-phenylpropylamine. *J. Pharmacol. Exp. Ther.,* 193:804–811, 1975.

Wong, D.T., & Yen, T.T. Suppression of appetite and reduction of body weight in normal and obese mice by fluoxetine, a selective inhibitor of serotonin uptake. *Fed. Proc.,* 44:1162, 1985.

Wurtman, J.J., Wurtman, R.J., Growdon, J., Henry, P., Lipscomb, A., & Zeisel, S. Carbohydrate craving in obese people: Suppression by treatments affecting serotoninergic transmission. *Int. J. Eat. Dis.,* 1:2–15, 1981.

Wurtman, J.J., Wurtman, R.J., Mark, S., Tsay, R., Gilbert, W., & Growdon, J. D-fenfluramine selectively suppresses carbohydrate snacking by obese subjects. *Int. J. Eat. Dis.,* 4:89–99, 1985.

Wurtman, J.J., Moses, P.L., & Wurtman, R.J. Prior carbohydrate consumption affects the amount of carbohydrate that rats choose to eat. *J. Nutr.,* 113:70–78, 1982.

Wurtman, J.J., & Wurtman, R.J. Fenfluramine and fluoxetine spare protein consumption while suppressing caloric intake by rats. *Sci.,* 198:1178–1180, 1977.

Wurtman, J.J., & Wurtman, R.J. Impaired control of appetite for carbohydrates in some patients with eating disorders: Treatment with pharmacological agents. In K.M. Pirke & D. Ploog (Eds.), *The Psychobiology of Anorexia Nervosa.* Berlin: Springer-Verlag, 1984a.

Wurtman, R.J., & Wurtman, J.J. Nutritional control of central neurotransmitters. In K.M. Pirke & D. Ploog (Eds.), *The Psychobiology of Anorexia Nervosa.* Berlin: Springer-Verlag, 1984b.

Young, S.N. Monoamine precursors in the affective disorders. *Adv. Hum. Psychopharmacol.,* 3:251–285, 1984.

8

Opioid Antagonist Drugs in the Treatment of Anorexia Nervosa

Walter H. Kaye

In the past decade studies on animals have found that opioid peptide systems endogenous to the brain contribute to the modulation of appetitive behavior (Morley & Levine, 1980; Sanger, 1981). These findings have led to speculation that disturbances of brain opioid peptides might be responsible for abnormal appetite or weight in humans (Givens, Wiedmann, Andersen, & Kitabchi, 1980; Margules, 1979; Margules, Moisset, Lewis, Shibuya, & Pert, 1978). In the past few years several studies have confirmed the existence of a disturbance of endogenous opioids in anorexia nervosa (Baranowska, Rozbicka, Jeske, & Abdec-Fatiah, 1984; Kaye, Berrettini, Gwirtsman, George, et al., 1986; Kaye, Pickar, Naber, & Ebert, 1982). Two preliminary studies (Luby, 1986, personal communication; Moore & Mills, 1981) using opioid antagonists (drugs that block opioid receptors) have raised the question of whether these drugs might provide beneficial treatment for patients with anorexia nervosa. It should be noted that the treatment of eating disorders with opioid medications is in its infancy and not enough data exist to recommend the use of opioid antagonists in the routine treatment of anorexia nervosa.

Because drugs that act on opioid systems are a theoretically promising avenue of treatment of anorexia nervosa, this chapter provides a brief overview of the relationship between endogenous opioid peptides and appetite regulation. Then studies demonstrating disturbances of endogenous opioids in anorexia nervosa are reviewed, and the chapter concludes with a review of the studies in which opioid antagonists are used to treat eating disorders. It is important to note that opioid antagonists have been found to decrease food intake in animal experiments (Brands, Thorhill, Hirst, & Gowdey, 1979; Frenk & Rogers, 1979; McCarthy, Dettman, Lynn, & Sanger, 1981; Recant, Voyles, Luciano, & Pert, 1980) as well as when given to healthy controls (Cohen, Cohen, Pickar, & Murphy, 1985) and obese human subjects (Atkinson, 1982; Wolkowitz, Doran, Cohen, Cohen, et al., 1985). These data from animal and normal and obese human studies suggest that opioid antagonists could produce effects on appetite that would be counterproductive for patients with anorexia nervosa.

RELATIONSHIP BETWEEN OPIOID PEPTIDES AND APPETITE REGULATION: OVERVIEW

Considerable data, derived primarily from animal experimentation, have suggested that endogenous opioid peptides are among the neurotransmitters that activate feeding behavior in the central nervous system (CNS). Although review of the relationship between endogenous opioid systems and appetitive behavior is beyond the scope of this chapter, a brief overview describing endogenous opioids and their relationship to feeding behavior might be useful for putting clinical studies into perspective.

At least three, and perhaps as many as five, separate families of opioid peptides exist in the brain, each having a discrete neuroanatomy (Bloom, 1983). A family of neuropeptides consists of several small sister neuropeptides that are derived from a mother precursor molecule. For example, beta-endorphin is derived from the precursor molecule pro-opiomelanocortin (POMC) (Krieger, Liotta, Brownstein, & Zimmerman, 1980). Other sister peptides that come from POMC include the N-terminal fragment of POMC adrenocorticotrophin hormone (ACTH), a peptide fragment located in the middle of the POMC precursor molecule; and beta-lipotropin, which forms the C-terminal end. Beta-endorphin is the C-terminal fragment of beta-lipotropin. To further complicate the picture, it has now been discovered that there are several derivatives of beta-endorphin and that these derivatives have various degrees of biologic activity.

The second family of opioids is derived from a large proenkephalin precursor molecule that produces both met- and leu-enkephalins. The third family of opioid neuropeptides produces dynorphins as well as other related opioid peptides. In addition to these three opioid peptide families, there appear to be other opioid peptides of uncertain parentage. Moreover, in addition to multiple endogenous opioid peptides, at least three different opioid receptor types have been discovered (Paterson, Robson, & Kosterlitz, 1983; Zukin & Zukin, 1981).

Early animal studies in this field presented an oversimplified picture of the relationship between endogenous opioids and appetitive behavior. Although it was clear that beta-endorphin and synthetic opioids such as morphine stimulated feeding behavior and that opioid antagonists reduced food intake, it has only been relatively recently discovered that the relationship between opioids and appetite is quite complicated. It is now recognized that several opioid peptides and receptors modulate feeding behavior. Morley, Levine, Gosnell, & Billington (1984) recently reviewed evidence that, in rats, the opioid peptide dynorphin, acting on the kappa opioid receptor, and the peptide beta-endorphin, acting on the epsilon opioid receptor, appeared to enhance feeding behavior. On the other hand, opioid systems may also inhibit food intake; for example, stimulation of the mu receptor system may decrease food intake.

In addition to brain-endogenous opioid systems that act on appetite centers, opioid peptides also play a role in modulating release of glucoregulatory hormones (Morley, 1983) from the pituitary (Grossman, 1983) and pancreas (Pfeiffer & Herz, 1984). If a drug, such as naloxone, were clinically effective in treating eating disorders, it might be because of the effects on the appetite centers in the hypothalamus or on hormones in the periphery that regulate the utilization of energy supplies by cells in the body. Either mechanism could alter food intake or the rate of weight gain.

DISTURBANCES OF BRAIN ENDOGENOUS OPIOIDS IN ANOREXIA NERVOSA

Anorexia nervosa is a disorder of unknown etiology distinguished by a fear of becoming obese and the relentless pursuit of thinness. The gratification shown by anorexics when refusing food and losing weight defies normal life-sustaining biologic drives. Anorexics' persistent self-starvation could be the result of a malfunction of the neurotransmitter systems known to modulate feeding behavior.

Results of several studies support the possibility that a disturbance of endogenous opioid activity exists in underweight, malnourished anorexics. An abnormal gonadotropin and pituitary adrenal response to a naloxone challenge has been reported in anorexia nervosa (Baranowska et al., 1984). Investigators have measured levels of opioids in cerebrospinal fluid (CSF), a method of directly estimating brain opioid production. Our group (Kaye et al., 1982) found underweight anorexics to have an increase in total opioid activity in CSF using a methodology that quantitated all compounds with opiate activity in CSF, and did not specify which opiate compounds were measured. CSF beta-endorphin in anorexic patients has been measured in two studies: Gerner and Sharp (1982) found anorexics to have normal levels of CSF beta-endorphin, whereas a recent study by our group (Kaye et al., 1986) found underweight anorexics to have reduced CSF beta-endorphin concentrations.

The results of these three CSF studies may seem contradictory, but several points will clarify the discrepancies. First, as described above, beta-endorphin is only one of many endogenous opioid peptides. In fact, beta-endorphin values (Kaye et al., 1986) were less than 1% of the value for total opioid activity in CSF determined by our earlier study (Kaye et al., 1982). Since several families of opioid peptides exist in the brain, elevated levels of one of a member of another family may have accounted for the increased total opioid activity found by the assay. Second, the patients studied by Gerner and Sharp (1982), although anorexic, had begun to refeed and gain weight. In contrast, we studied patients who were still very much malnourished (Kaye et al., 1986). Furthermore, we found a positive correlation between CSF beta-endorphin concentrations and caloric intake ($p < .05$) in low-weight anorexics. Together these data suggest that reduced beta-endorphin levels are associated with malnutrition in anorexia nervosa and that CSF beta-endorphin levels can be rapidly raised by improved nutrition, even before much weight gain.

Alterations in opioid peptides in anorexia nervosa normalize after weight is gained (Kaye et al., 1982; Kaye et al., 1986) and thus are most likely secondary to weight loss and starvation. Until prospective studies in anorexia nervosa are conducted, it is impossible to know whether disturbed opioid function does in fact drive this illness. Whether disturbances in opioid function in anorexia nervosa are intrinsic to anorexia nervosa or secondary to weight loss, disturbances in brain opioid pathways may still be contributing to other symptoms found in malnourished anorexics such as neuroendocrine dysregulation.

USE OF OPIOID ANTAGONISTS IN TREATING EATING DISORDERS: REVIEWS OF STUDIES

In a study by Moore and Mills (1981), underweight patients with anorexia nervosa received continuous intravenous infusions of naloxone (3.2 to 6.4 mg/day) for an average of five weeks in the midst of being refed and gaining weight. Patients were reported to gain significantly more weight in the week following the start of the naloxone infusion compared with the week prior to beginning the naloxone infusion and the week after the naloxone was stopped. This study was conducted to demonstrate that naloxone had an antilipolytic effect in humans (plasma beta-hydroxybutyrate and nonesterified fatty acid levels fell during the infusion). It was reported that the anorexics gained more weight while they were on naloxone than they did when they were not taking naloxone even though their caloric intake was the same either off or on the drug. (The actual caloric intake consumed by anorexics, however, was not reported.)

Several methodologic problems with this study question whether naloxone is therapeutically useful in anorexics. First, for the most part, Moore and Mills (1981) did not blind the patients or the staff (two patients were reported to get a brief trial of saline under single-blind conditions). Thus, there may have been a considerable placebo effect to a prolonged IV infusion. Second, patients were also taking amitriptyline during this study, which might have contributed to any beneficial responses. Finally, Gillman and Lichtigfeld (1981) raised the possibility that the weight-gain effect of naloxone in the study by Moore and Mills (1981) was the result of the drug's inhibition of vomiting.

Another opioid antagonist, naltrexone, has been given to five anorexic patients (Luby, personal communication, 1986) in preliminary open trial done on inpatients in an eating-disorder program. Each subject had been admitted after substantial weight loss and was given naltrexone (75 to 100 mg/day orally in divided doses) while concurrently in a refeeding and weight-gaining program. Three of the patients (two women, one man) were in their thirties and had been ill with anorexia nervosa for five years or longer. These subjects gained 20 to 40 pounds of weight on naltrexone. Most interestingly, each continued to take the naltrexone after discharge and each was reported to have maintained his or her weight on follow-up, eight to 12 months after discharge. Two patients, however, failed to respond to naltrexone. These two patients were teenage women who had been ill with anorexia nervosa for less than four years. One of these patients gained 15 pounds and then refused to take any more naltrexone; the other patient did not gain any weight on this medication.

Since this is a preliminary and open trial, the findings should be viewed with caution. Whereas many open trial, nonblind case reports have claimed that a variety of medications are an effective treatment for anorexia nervosa, such findings have not been substantiated by more rigorous methodology. It is of interest, however, that the older, more chronic patients were the ones that appeared to benefit from naltrexone. In general, older chronic patients are often the most resistant to treatment.

In direct contrast to the studies cited above, in which opiate antagonists have been reported to increase weight gain in underweight anorexics, opiate antagonists have been found to reduce food intake in animal experiments (Brands et al., 1979; Frenk & Rogers, 1979; McCarthy et al., 1981; Recant et al., 1980) and when given to normal and obese human subjects. Naloxone was found to decrease food intake in healthy control subjects in a study by Cohen et al. (1985). Food intake from two meals following a single naloxone infusion (2 mg/kg) was significantly reduced compared with food intake following a placebo infusion in double-blind crossover conditions. In a study by Atkinson (1982), obese humans and controls received an infusion of either one of two doses (2 or 15 mg) of naloxone or of saline. Atkinson found that food intake decreased with a 15 mg naloxone infusion in obese humans but not in lean controls or in obese humans given 2 mg of naloxone. Wolkowitz et al. (1985) gave naloxone (0.5 mg/kg by intravenous injection) to six obese subjects in a double blind study. Subjects were given either naloxone or placebo after an overnight fast. Food consumption during lunch and dinner was measured. Subjects ate 25% less food on the day they received naloxone.

SUMMARY

Although considerable animal data suggest that opioid pathways are important contributors to the regulation of appetite and a number of studies suggest that opioid activity is disturbed in underweight anorexics, it is not clear that opioid antagonists such as naloxone or naltrexone are useful in the treatment of anorexia nervosa. There are a number of reasons for not making such a conclusion at this time. First, the few trials that have been conducted so far have involved few subjects and have been uncontrolled. Thus, it remains unclear whether the reported weight-gain effects were a response to the drug or to suggestion.

Moreover, considerable animal data and a few studies in obese and lean humans have found that naloxone reduces food intake. Such strong and consistently replicated data suggest that opioid antagonists would be counterproductive in treating anorexics. Even in the face of these data, it is still possible that anorexics could have a paradoxical response to opioid antagonists. This is because opioid antagonists act, to a different degree, on more than one of the opioid receptors. As was explained in the overview, it has been learned that multiple opioid neuropeptides and receptors exist in humans. Limited data suggest that the normal balance of these peptides (and perhaps receptors) is altered in anorexia nervosa. Therefore, it is difficult to predict how anorexics would respond to any opioid drug.

If opioid antagonists were found to produce beneficial weight gain in anorexia nervosa, many unanswered issues would still attend its use. For one, it is not known whether prolonged administration of opiate antagonists to underweight anorexics is harmful. In addition, naloxone requires intravenous infusion, a considerable problem in the chronic treatment of any patient. It is important to note that the dose of nalaxone given by Moore and Mills (1981) was much lower than the dose used in controls and obese human studies. If investigators are tempted to use higher doses of naloxone in anorexia nervosa, they should be aware that higher doses of naloxone can produce behavioral, hormonal, and physiological effects (such as changes in blood pressure) in healthy controls (Cohen, Cohen, Pickar, Weingartner, & Murphy, 1983). Thus, higher doses of naloxone in anorexia nervosa might produce dangerous alterations in autonomic function and the possibility of destabilization of mood.

The relationship between opioid function and appetite is a rapidly advancing area of research, and with this advance more specific drugs are becoming available that may facilitate treatment of eating disorders. Much more research is required, however, before opioid-antagonizing drugs should be used routinely to treat anorexia nervosa.

REFERENCES

Atkinson, R. L. Naloxone decreases food intake in obese humans. *J. Clin. Endo. Metab.*, 55:196–198, 1982.

Baranowska, B., Rozbicka, G., Jeske, W., & Abdec-Fatiah, M. H. The role of endogenous opiates in the mechanism of inhibited luteinizing hormone (LH) secretion in women with anorexia nervosa: The effect of naloxone of LH, follicle-stimulating hormone, prolactin, and beta-endorphin secretion. *J. Clin. Endo. Metab.*, 59:412–416, 1984.

Bloom, R. E. The endorphins: A growing family of pharmacologically pertinent peptides. *Ann. Rev. Pharmacol. Toxicol.*, 23:151–170, 1983.

Brands, B., Thorhill, J. A., Hirst, M., & Gowdey, C. W. Suppression of food intake and body weight gain by naloxone in rats. *Life Sci.*, 24:1773–1778, 1979.

Cohen, M. R., Cohen, R. M., Pickar, D., Weingartner, H., & Murphy, D. L. High dose naloxone infusions in normals. *Arch. Gen. Psychiatry*, 40:613–619, 1983.

Cohen, M. R., Cohen, R. M., Pickar, D., & Murphy, D. L. Naloxone reduces food intake in humans. *Psychosomat. Med.*, 47:132–137, 1985.

Frenk, J., & Rogers, G. H. The suppressant effects of naloxone on food

and water intake in the rat. *Behav. and Neural Biol.,* 26:23-40, 1979.
Gerner, R. H., & Sharp, B. CSF beta-endorphin-immunoreactivity in normal, schizophrenic, depressed, manic and anorexia subjects. *Brain Res.,* 237:244-247, 1982.
Gillman, M. A., & Lichtigfeld, F. J. Naloxone in anorexia nervosa: Role of the opiate system. *J. Roy. Soc. Med.,* 74:631-632, 1981.
Givens, J. R., Wiedmann, E., Andersen, R. N., & Kitabchi, A. E. Beta-endorphin and beta-lipotropin plasma levels in hirsute women: Correlation with body weight. *J. Clin. Endo. Metab.,* 50:975-976, 1980.
Grossman, A. Brain opiates and neuroendocrine functions. *Clinics Endocrinol. Metab.,* 12:725-746, 1983.
Kaye, W. H., Pickar, D., Naber, D., & Ebert, M. H. Cerebrospinal fluid opioid activity in anorexia nervosa. *J. Psych.,* 139:643-645, 1982.
Kaye, W. H., Berrettini, W. H., Gwirtsman, H. E., George, T., Jimerson, D. C., & Gold, P. W. Alterations of CSF, CRH, and POMC in anorexia nervosa. Paper presented at the American Psychiatric Association 139th Annual Meeting, Washington, D.C., May 1986.
Krieger, D. T., Liotta, A. S., Brownstein, M. J., & Zimmerman, E. A. ACTH, beta-lipotropin, and related peptides in brain, pituitary, and blood. *Recent Prog. Horm. Res.,* 36:277-344, 1980.
Luby, E. Personal communication. Harper Grace Hospitals, Detroit, Michigan, 1986.
Margules, D. L., Moisset, B., Lewis, M. J., Shibuya, H., & Pert, C. B. Beta-endorphin is associated with overeating in genetically obese mice (ob/ob) and rats (fa/fa). *Science,* 202:988-991, 1978.
Margules, D. L. The obesity of middle age: A common variety of Cushing's syndrome due to a chronic increase in adrenocorticotrophin (ACTH) and beta-endorphin activity. *Neuro. Behav. Rev.,* 3:107-111, 1979.
McCarthy, P. S., Dettman, P. W., Lynn, A. G., & Sanger, D. J. Anorectic actions of the opiate antagonist naloxone. *Neuropharmacol.,* 20:1347-1349, 1981.
Moore, R., & Mills, I. H. Naloxone in the treatment of anorexia nervosa: Effect on weight gain and lipolysis. *J. Roy. Soc. Med.,* 74:129-131, 1981.
Morley, J. E. Neuroendocrine effects of endogenous opioid peptides in human subjects: A review. *Psychoneuroendocrinol.,* 8(4):361-379, 1983.

Morley, J. E., & Levine, A. S. Stress-induced eating is mediated through endogenous opiates. *Science,* 209:1259–1261, 1980.

Morley, J. E., Levine, A. S., Gosnell, B. A., & Billington, C. J. Which opioid receptor mechanism modulates feeding? *Appetite,* 5:61–68, 1984.

Paterson, S. J., Robson, L. E., & Kosterlitz, H. W. Classification of opioid receptor. *Brit. Med. Bull.,* 39:31–36, 1983.

Pfeiffer, A., & Herz, A. Endocrine actions of opioids. *Horm. Met. Res.,* 16:386–397, 1984.

Recant, L., Voyles, N. R., Luciano, M., & Pert, C. B. Naltrexone reduces weight gain, alters "beta-endorphin," and reduces insulin output from pancreatic islets of genetically obese mice. *Peptides,* 1:309–313, 1980.

Sanger, D. J. Endorphinergic mechanisms in the control of food and water intake. *Appetite: J. Intake Res.,* 2:193–208, 1981.

Stapleton, J. M., Lind, M. D., Merriman, V. J., & Reid, L. D. Naloxone inhibits diazepam-induced feeding in rats. *Life Sci.,* 24:2421–2425, 1979.

Wolkowitz, O. M., Doran, A. R., Cohen, M. R., Cohen, R. M., Wise, T. N., & Pickar, D. Effect of naloxone on food consumption in obesity. *New Eng. J. Med.,* 313:327, 1985.

Zukin, R. S., & Zukin, S. R. Multiple opiatereceptors: Emerging concepts. *Life Sci.,* 29:2681–2690, 1981.

9

Drugs That Facilitate Gastric Emptying

Gerry Craigen, Sidney Kennedy, Paul E. Garfinkel, and Khursheed Jeejeebhoy

Patients with anorexia nervosa frequently complain of a number of gastrointestinal symptoms. These include nausea, regurgitation, early satiety, epigastric pain, abdominal distension, and vomiting. Acute gastric dilatation rarely has been described on refeeding (Evans, 1968; Russell, 1966). It is not known for certain what contributes to this early satiety and dyspepsia. On the one hand, when patients with anorexia nervosa were given a standard calorie load disguised into what appeared to be either a "high" or "low" calorie meal, their subjective ratings of satiety were greater after they had ingested the presumed high-calorie meal (Garfinkel, Moldofsky, & Garner, 1978), suggesting at least some conative component to their experience of satiety. On the other hand, there is considerable evidence that the above symptoms are related to a delay in gastric emptying. This chapter outlines mechanisms that are responsible for

---

We are grateful to Dr. Gordon Greenburg for advice, Brenda Lediett and Carrol Whynot for technical assistance in preparing this chapter, and to Patricia Thompson (Janssen Pharmaceutica) for domperidone.

This work was supported by the Canadian Psychiatric Research Foundation (Dr. S. Kennedy).

the control of gastric emptying, reviews findings of abnormal gastric functioning in anorexia nervosa, and describes the use of drugs to enhance gastric emptying in these patients.

CONTROL OF GASTRIC EMPTYING

Several mechanisms are involved in the control of gastric emptying. Physical and chemical, neurohormonal, and emotional factors are interconnected through a system of feedback loops (see Figure 9-1).

Chemical and Physical Control Factors

Food entering the duodenum affects gastric emptying through osmotic pressure effects. Fats, proteins, and carbohydrates all appear to slow gastric emptying equally in proportion to their calories, suggesting it is the shared nutrient value that is the important regulator of gastric emptying (Brener, Hendrix, & McHugh, 1983). Acidic solutions slow gastric emptying; higher acid concentrations cause greater inhibitory effects than lower acid concentrations (Hunt & Know, 1972). Reflex nervous signals are transmitted from the duodenum back to the stomach, which influences the tone of the pylorus and thus gastric emptying (Enterogastric Reflex). The Enterogastric (EG) Reflex is elicited by a number of factors including distension of the duodenum, acidity of chyme, and the fat and protein content of the chyme. The hormonal feedback from the duodenum to the stomach and the EG reflex work together to slow gastric emptying when too much chyme is in the small intestine or chyme is excessively acidic, contains too much fat or protein, is hypotonic or hypertonic, or is irritating to the duodenum. In this way the rate of stomach emptying is limited to the amount of chyme that the small intestine can process (Guyton, 1986).

Gastric distension has also been recognized as a potent satiety signal inhibiting food intake (Cannon & Washburn, 1912). How-

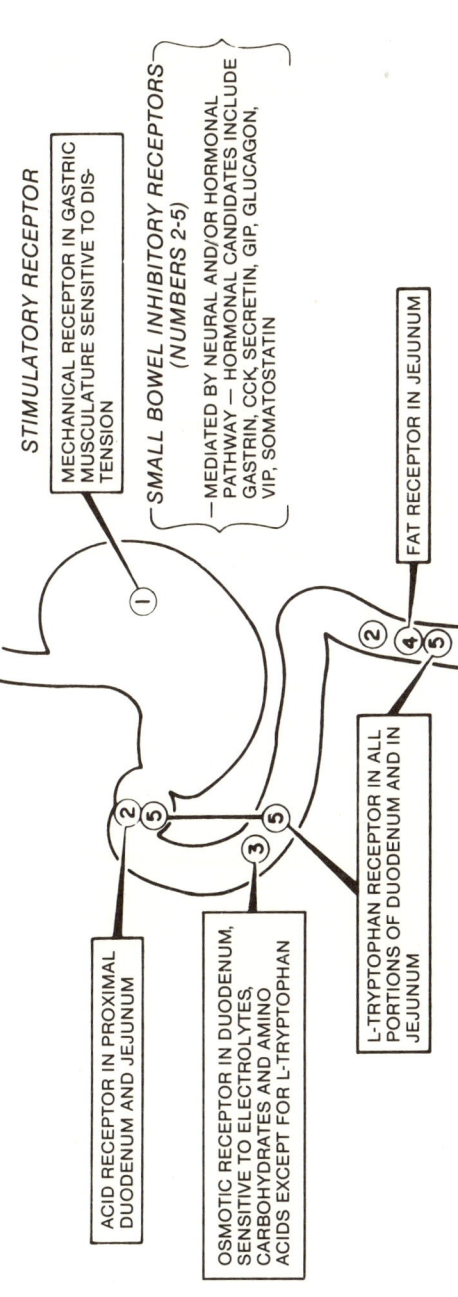

Figure 9-1. Physiology of gastric emptying. Various factors that influence gastric emptying are depicted. Location of mechanical and osmotic receptors (1 and 3) as determined by human studies. Other receptors localized by studies in dogs. Abbreviations: CCK, cholecystokinin; GIP, gastric inhibitory polypeptide; VIP, Vasoactive intestinal polypeptide. (Reprinted with permission from Minami & McCallum, 1984.)

ever, as McHugh and Moran (1985) state, distension could be viewed as a result of two events: the ingestion of food, and the inhibition of gastric emptying to facilitate digestion. This inhibition is caused by nutrients entering the small bowel that activates various feedback loops to the stomach which then inhibit further emptying. The primary determinant of emptying of liquids from the stomach is volume. There is a linear relationship between the rate of liquid emptying and intragastric pressure (Strunz & Grossman, 1978). On the other hand, in the intact stomach emptying of solids is dependent upon other factors such as particle size and antral motility (Meyer, Ohashi, Jehn, & Thompson, 1981).

Although thermostatic control mechanisms also contribute to food intake, there are at present no good data to implicate changes in overall body temperature in the control of human eating gastric emptying (Garfinkel & Coscina, 1982).

Neurohormonal Mechanisms of Control

The mechanisms by which gastric contents regulate their own emptying involve a network of sensors in the duodenal mucosa. Stimulation of these chemoreceptors slows gastric emptying (Ross, 1978). The pyloric sphincter is a zone of elevated pressure between the stomach and the gut which can contract further and reduce emptying. However, it is not entirely clear whether the tone of the sphincter is responsible for delayed gastric emptying. The alternative explanation is that gastric emptying is dependent upon the pressure gradient between the antrum and the duodenum as well as aboral propagation of pressure waves. When gastric acid and lipids contact the duodenal mucosa, the hormones secretin, gastric inhibitory peptide (GIP), and cholecystokinin (CCK) are released, and slow gastric emptying follows (Ross, 1978).

Vagal excitation causes release of gastrin and increases gastric emptying; emptied gastric contents stimulate release of secretin, enterogastrone, and CCK and activate mucosal receptors in the duodenum (see Figure 9-2). The four hormones act to decrease dis-

Drugs That Facilitate Gastric Emptying

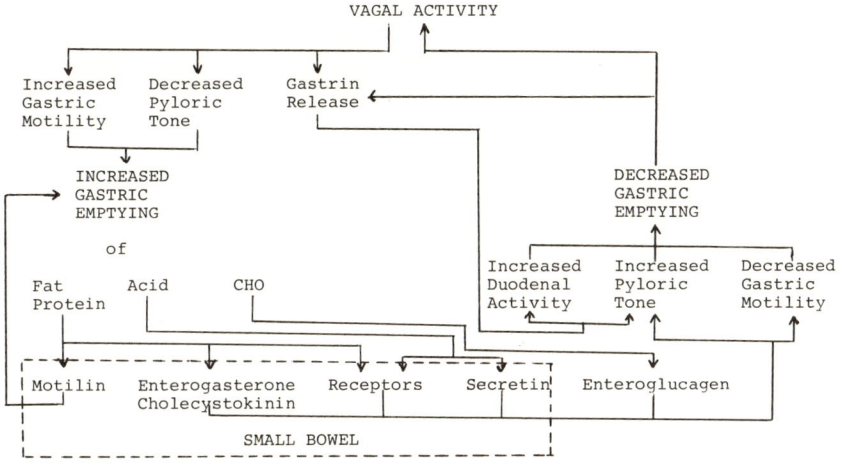

Figure 9-2. Control of gastric emptying. Nervous and hormonal factors operate as negative feedback to decrease gastric emptying after emptying has been stimulated.

tal stomach motility, increase pyloric tone, and increase duodenal motility that results in delayed gastric emptying (Ross, 1978).

McHugh and Moran (1985) have studied CCK in some detail. Using saline exchanges, they found that the stomach emptied rapidly before a CCK infusion, but an inhibition in its emptying was apparent immediately on beginning the hormone infusion and by the second exchange of saline, emptying had essentially ceased. Also when the hormone infusion was discontinued, there was immediate recovery of gastric emptying of the saline. The authors refer to this inhibitory effect on the stomach as a kind of endocrine square wave that suggests a role for CCK, a hormone of brief half-life, in switching on and off gastric emptying. At present the relationship of CCK to other inhibitory factors and the relationship of calories in the small intestine to the stimulation of CCK is unknown, but a major stimulus for CCK release is the presence of fat in the lumen of the gut (Bennett & McMartin, 1978). GIP may also have an inhibitory effect on gastric motility (Dixon, Zip, O'Dorisio, & Cataland, in press). Motilin is another hormone that also may affect gastric motility (Thomas, Kelly, & Go, 1979).

Specific neural mechanisms exist also to control gastric emptying. There are interconnections between the vagus nerve and the gut hormonal feedback (see Figure 9-2). The rate of gastric emptying is controlled both by cholinergic activity mediated through the vagus nerve and by dopamine (Valenzuela, 1976) and provides the rationale for the use of cholinergic and dopaminergic drugs to increase gastric emptying. Enkephalins may also play a role (Edin, Lundberg, Terenius, Dahlstrom, et al., 1980; Lundberg, Horfelt, Kewenter, Petterson, et al., 1979).

The gastrointestinal tract is much more active in secreting hormones than previously thought. A number of hormones are located both in the gut and in the brain. This has given rise to the concept of a gut brain axis. Hormones shared by the brain and by the gut include CCK, somatostatin, thyrotrophin-releasing hormone, and adrenocorticotrophin (Track, 1980). To what extent alterations in circulating levels of these hormones result from, rather than cause, gastric disturbances is of current research interest.

Emotional Factors Involved in Gastric Emptying

The possibility that gastric emptying may be altered in emotional disturbances was first suggested by Cannon in 1898. Stress may indirectly delay gastric motility by increasing acid secretion. A direct effect on the sympathetic nervous system (through the fight or flight response) may also occur. Strong sympathetic stimulation inhibits peristalsis and increases the tone of the sphincters. The net result is greatly slowed propulsion of food throughout the G.I. tract (Guyton, 1986). The fact that central dopaminergic inhibition by metoclopramide can increase the rate of gastric emptying suggests that alterations in central neurotransmitter levels may alter gastric motility (Costall, Gunning, Naylor, & Simpson, 1983). As far as we are aware, other emotional factors involved in gastric emptying have not been worked out in terms of their direct relationship to specific nervous system mechanisms.

DISTURBANCES OF GASTRIC EMPTYING IN PATIENTS WITH EATING DISORDERS

A number of techniques have been introduced to measure gastric emptying. These may involve (a) intubation, (b) radiological assessment, or (c) radioisotope scanning. Earlier studies of gastric motility using barium meal and continuous gastric infusion techniques failed to show any major abnormality in anorexia nervosa patients (Scobie, 1973; Silverstone & Russell, 1967). Subsequently, Dubois and associates (1979) using a gastric intubation technique reported a delay in gastric emptying in patients with anorexia nervosa. Following weight gain these values tended to return toward the control values. However, the effect of gastric intubation may in itself account for altered gastric motility. However, since liquid emptying is related to gastric tone and solid emptying is related to antral contractions, these studies cannot determine the changes in the emptying of solids. They only examine liquid emptying. More recently, several authors have used isotope techniques to measure solid and liquid emptying times in patients with anorexia nervosa compared to controls.

Holt and associates (1981) used a scintiscanning technique to study simultaneous liquid and solid emptying in 10 female anorexic patients and 12 controls. All of the patient group had at some time complained of early satiety, postprandial discomfort, or recurrent vomiting. Significantly slower gastric emptying was found for both liquid and solid components of the test meal in the anorexic group, although emptying during the early phase (0–10 minutes after meal ingestion) was not significantly different in the two groups. The authors suggest this may reflect normal vagal-mediated postprandial receptive relaxation in anorexia nervosa. Using a similar technique McCallum and colleagues (1985) reported on gastric emptying in 16 low-weight anorexics and 13 asymptomatic normal-weight controls. Solid emptying was significantly slower in the anorexic group, but liquid emptying was similar in both groups. Since the antrum is mainly responsible for emptying of solids (Wilbur & Kelly, 1973), the authors suggest that either a primary or secondary disturbance in antral motility occurs in anorexia nervosa. A third group (Saleh & Lebwohl, 1980) also demonstrated delayed gastric emptying in seven anorexic patients, whereas Stacher and associates (1985a) reported gross delay in gastric emptying of a semisolid test meal in six of 10 anorexics and both of two bulimic subjects. ($T1/2$ ranged from 117–193 minutes compared to 52.9 ± 4.3 minutes as the mean $T1/2$ for 24 healthy controls.) This same group (Stacher, Kiss, Wiesnagrotzki, Bergmann, et al., 1985b) also reported a significant esophageal motility disorder in 30% of patients with anorexia nervosa.

More recently, tentative evidence has emerged suggesting a link between an increased GIP response to meal stimulation in low-weight anorexics and delayed gastric emptying (Dixon, Zip, O'Dorisio, & Cataland, 1985). However, this finding was not confirmed by Nelson and Solyom (1985), who reported a lower GIP response to a liquid test meal in anorexic patients compared to bulimics and normal controls.

In summary, a number of studies over the past decade have recorded delayed gastric emptying times (especially for solids) among people with anorexia nervosa. Corresponding studies on bulimic patients at present are confined to a few case reports. The mechanisms responsible for the delay in emptying are not clearly understood, but recent developments in understanding the gut-brain axis suggest a possible bridging role for such hormones as GIP and CCK.

DRUGS THAT FACILITATE GASTRIC EMPTYING

Since gastric emptying is controlled by a sequence of interacting mechanisms (see Figure 9-2), it is not surprising that several drugs with differing pharmacological effects all produce gastrokinetic effects. Bethanecol, a cholinergic agent, decreases the frequency and duration of reflux episodes and increases lower esophageal sphincter pressure (Euler, 1980). Metoclopramide, a potent dopamine antagonist with central nervous system and gastrointestinal effects, increases gastric and duodenal peristalsis in children (Hitch, Vanhoutte, & Torres-Pinedo, 1982). It also accelerates gastric emptying in adult patients with gastroesophageal reflux and delayed gastric emptying (McCallum, Fink, Lerner, & Berkowitz, 1983). Domperidone is a potent peripheral dopamine antagonist with less cholinergic activity than metoclopramide; it does not appear to cross the blood-brain barrier and hence produces fewer neurological side effects. Domperidone is also an effective gastrokinetic agent (Brogden, Carmine, Heel, Speight, & Avery, 1982), although its effects on esophageal motility are less clear (Grill, Hilemeier, Semeraro, McCallum, & Gryboski, 1985). Cisapride, an acetylcholine release-enhancing compound without dopamine antagonistic properties, also appears to have gastrokinetic properties (Schuurkes & Van Nueten, 1984).

These four drugs were compared according to their ability to improve antroduodenal coordination, which McCallum and associates (1985) postulated to be disturbed in anorexia nervosa (Schuurkes & Van Nueten, 1984). They found that domperidone and cisapride, and to a lesser extent metoclopramide but not bethanecol, were found to effectively improve antroduodenal coordination, which supports a role for both dopaminergic and cholinergic pathways in controlling gastric emptying.

A number of the above investigations of gastric emptying in anorexic patients (Dubois, Gross, Richter, & Ebert, 1981; McCallum, Grill, Lange, Planky, et al., 1985; Saleh & Lebwohl, 1980) also reported on the acute effect on gastric emptying following a single dose infusion of one of these drugs. Saleh and Lebwohl (1980) found a return to normal gastric emptying in three of four anorexic patients with delayed emptying after oral ingestion of 10 mg of metoclopramide 30 minutes before repeat testing. Although patients continued to take metoclopramide 10 mg before each meal and at bedtime with reported subjective benefit, no further evaluation of gastric emptying was documented, nor was there a critical evaluation of the clinical benefit of metoclopramide in an ongoing fashion.

McCallum and associates (1985) also reported on the beneficial effect of a single intramuscular injection of metoclopramide 10 mg in a group of anorexic patients with a previously documented delay in gastric emptying of solids. In nine of the 11 subjects, there was more than a 10% decrease in isotope retained in the stomach after 120 minutes.

Dubois and colleagues (1981), using the same gastric intubation technique previously described (Dubois, Gross, Ebert, & Castell, 1979), reported on the effect of a single subcutaneous injection of bethanecol (0.06 mg/kg) on gastric acid output and fractional emptying rates. This acute cholinergic stimulation temporarily increased gastric acid output and fractional emptying threefold in both anorexic and control groups. However, the authors did not treat their patients with bethanecol on an ongoing basis. Similarly, Stacher and colleagues (1985a) under double-blind conditions reported a significant improvement in gastric emptying following a 10 mg intravenous injection of cisapride in 10 anorexic and two bulimic patients. ($T1/2$ on cisapride was 44.7 ± 5.0 minutes as compared to 115.8 ± 13.5 minutes with intravenous saline placebo; $p < .001$.)

This literature clearly documents the benefits of acute administration of antidopaminergic or cholinergic agents on the delayed gastric emptying of anorexia nervosa, but does not deal with potential benefit from longer-term administration.

Two preliminary studies question whether there is an ongoing role for metoclopramide and domperidone in the treatment of satiety symptoms and dyspepsia in anorexia nervosa. Moldofsky and colleagues (1977) reported on five anorexic patients who took part in a four-week placebo-controlled study of metoclopramide. Although there was a strong subjective sense of relief of gastrointestinal symptoms, drug-induced depression prevented two of the five patients from continuing to take the drug. Moreover, since metoclopramide is a potent dopamine blocker which crosses the blood-brain barrier, there is a significant risk of neurological and motor side effects including tardive dyskinesia (Grimes, Hassan, & Preston, 1982; Wiholm, Mortimer, Boethius, & Haggstrom, 1984). For this reason, interest has shifted to domperidone. In a single case report, Russell and associates (1983) found that domperidone improved subjective ratings of satiety and after 14 days shortened gastric emptying time for solids from 119 minutes to 75 minutes.

As a consequence of this, we have carried out a double-blind placebo-controlled crossover study of domperidone in female patients admitted to the Inpatient Eating Disorder Service at Toronto General Hospital who, in addition to a DSM-III diagnosis of anorexia nervosa (not necessarily currently 25% below ideal body weight), have at least one complaint related to altered gastric emptying, including early satiety, bloating, fullness after meals, or vomiting.

After an informed consent was obtained, the patients proceeded into a six-week study; two weeks of observation (washout), and four weeks on a double-blind placebo-controlled, randomized crossover trial of domperidone 20 mg p.o. t.i.d., given 30 minutes before meals. Immediately after meals, and after further intervals of 20 and 60 minutes, the patients rated their symptom state of fullness on a 10 cm analog scale and also recorded whether nausea or vomiting was present. At two-week intervals (after washout, placebo, and drug), sequential gastric scintiscanning was carried out using the technique described by Coates and associates (1973). Satiety questionnaires were completed and weights were recorded (see Figure 9-3).

Of 14 consecutive admissions who met the above criteria, 10 agreed to undergo the study and nine completed the study. One patient signed out of the hospital against medical advice during the washout period. Three patients who had previously taken tricyclic antidepressants continued to take these during the study. Apart from domperidone, all other patients were drug-free before and during the study (see Table 9-1).

Mean visual analog scores after each meal at three time points (0, 20, and 60 minutes) showed no significant benefit for domperidone over placebo, although both showed improvement over the washout phase (see Figure 9-4). There was a nonsignificant trend toward

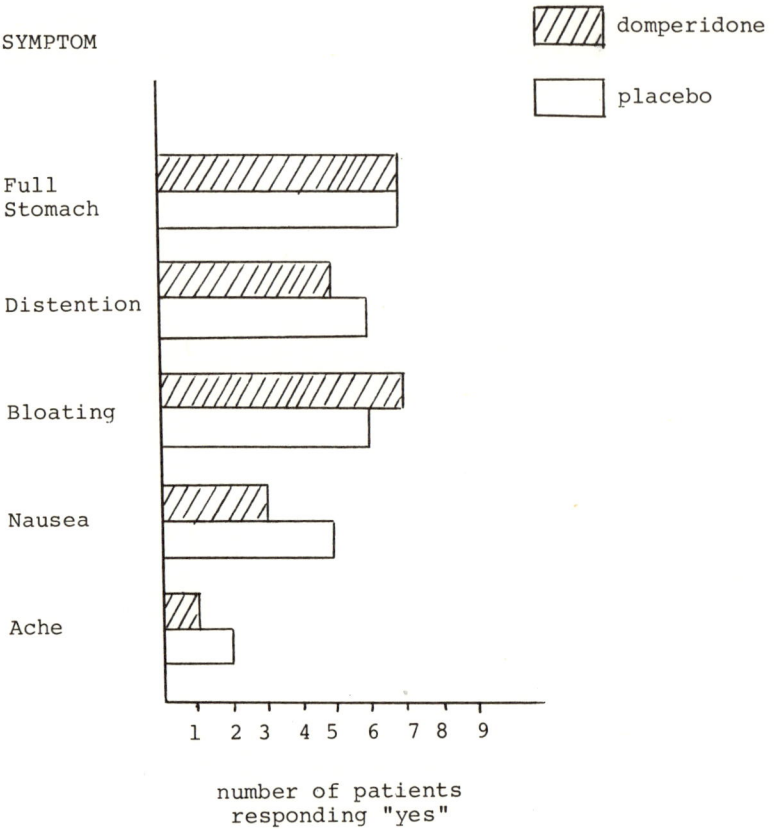

Figure 9-3. Subjective reports of satiety after 14 days of treatment on domperidone and placebo.

improvement in nausea ratings on domperidone as compared to both washout and placebo phases. Similarly, gastric emptying did not improve during either domperidone or placebo compared to the washout phase (see Figure 9-5). Results expressed as $T1/2$ for each phase of solid emptying were as follows: washout 76.6 ± 16.5 minutes; domperidone 74.9 ± 19.2 minutes; and placebo 79.7 ± 13.2 minutes. Their rate of emptying of liquid from the stomach was normal during washout and drug phases.

Table 9-1

Patients with Anorexia Nervosa Who
Completed Domperidone Study (N = 9)

	Means
Age (yrs.)	29.8 ± 5.8
Duration of illness (yrs.)	5.5 ± 2.4
Height (cm)	161.0 ± 6.7
Weight at start (kg)	45.1 ± 8.1
%IBW at start (kg)	78.1 ± 9.9
Weight after domperidone (kg)	45.9 ± 4.8
%IBW after domperidone (kg)	81.5 ± 8.9
Weight after placebo (kg)	48.3 ± 7.5
%IBW after placebo (kg)	83.8 ± 7.8

Plasma levels of domperidone drawn at the end of the 14-day period of active drug treatment are so far available for the first six subjects. These reflect steady-state and two-hour postingestion peak values (see Table 9-2).

Initial results from this trial suggest that domperidone is not useful in an ongoing fashion for patients with anorexia nervosa who, in addition, experience subjective bloating and fullness. However, there are several lines of inquiry that should be pursued before reaching any firm conclusions.

It is interesting to note that patient #3 who showed the most marked improvement also had the highest plasma levels of domperidone. In view of the low oral bioavailability of domperidone, reported by Heykants and colleagues (1981), it is possible that the

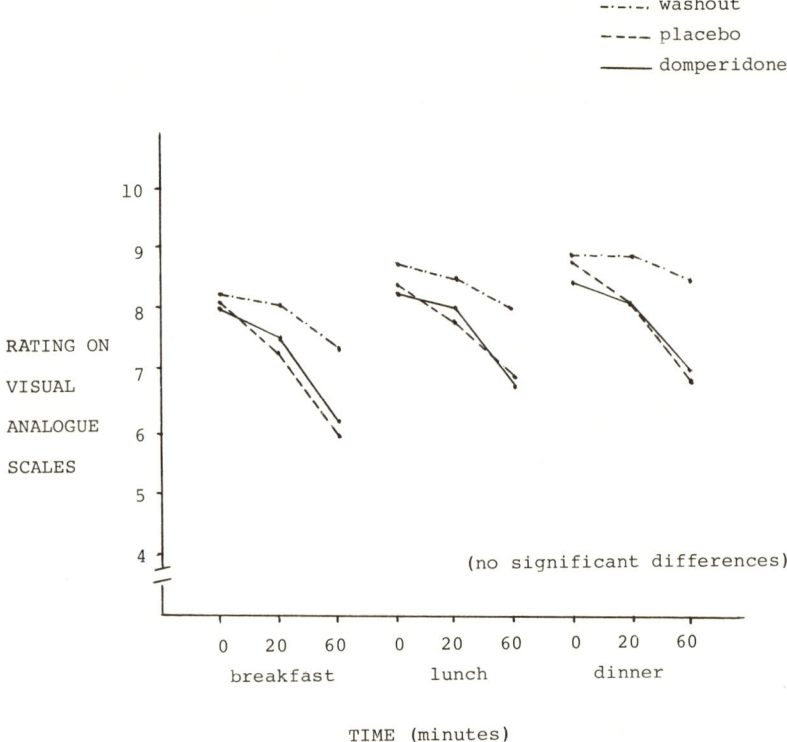

Figure 9-4. Visual analogue ratings of satiety at three time points after meals during washout, placebo, and domperidone phases.

majority of the patients were in fact underdosed. However, the prescribed dosage of 20 mg three times daily, 30 minutes before meals is the currently recommended regimen. It should also be noted that patients were selected for this study based on subjective symptoms reported and not initial delay in solid gastric emptying. This resulted in a group being studied who did not, in fact, show an abnormality in gastric emptying time at the preliminary assessment (mean $T1/2$ solid 76.7 ± 16.5 minutes—normal range 60–90 minutes). Perhaps only those individuals with a documented delay in gastric emptying (especially for solids) should be selected for

Drugs That Facilitate Gastric Emptying

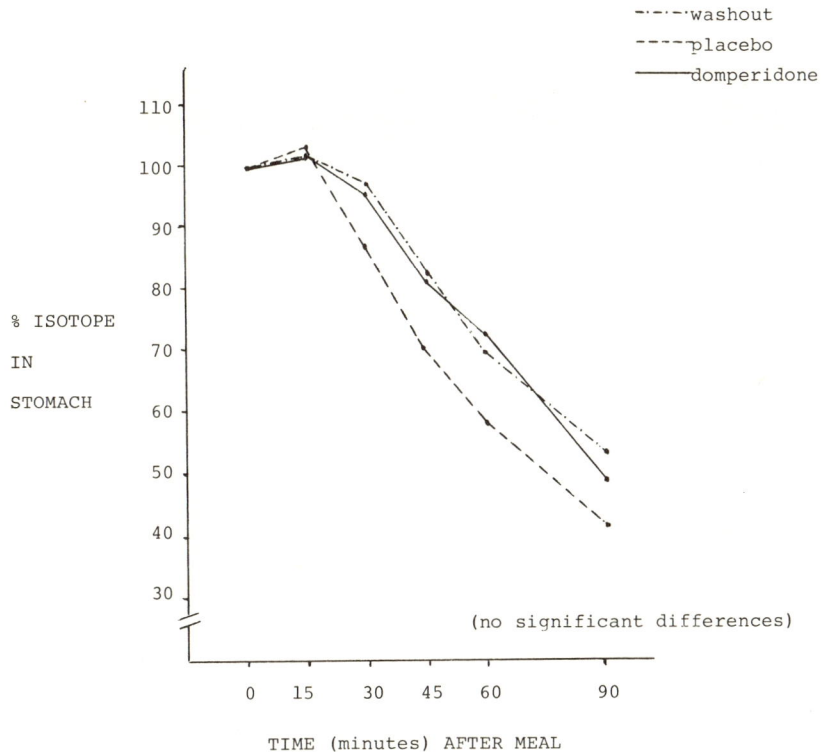

Figure 9-5. Gastric emptying of solids expressed as % isotope remaining in stomach at 15-minute intervals for 90 minutes after ingestion of solid phase marker.

study of the medication. It is also difficult to assess precisely what the visual analog scale of satiety measures. A body image distortion and relentless pursuit of thinness may impair the ability to rate change in gastric distension, particularly if it is associated with expectations that more food will be consumed leading to weight gain. Side effects were not significant during this brief study. One patient developed galactorrhea, which stopped on discontinuing medication. Domperidone does not appear to cross the blood-brain barrier, but its use on a long-term basis would be of some concern.

Table 9-2

Plasma Levels of Domperidone after 14-Day Trial Showing Steady State and Two-Hour Postingestion Peak Levels

Patient #	T 1/2 SOLID			PLASMA DOMPERIDONE	
	Washout	Domperidone	Placebo	Time 1	Time 2
1	>90	>90	>90	4.4	18.8
2	56	42	89	2.9	12.8
3*	>90	57	>90	4.0	20.3
4	53	64	76	3.2	4.0
5	73	73	55	4.0	8.3
6	>90	>90	75	3.9	9.0

*Concurrently received amitriptyline 150 mg daily.

SUMMARY

In conclusion, several reports have confirmed a delay in gastric emptying among anorexic patients, particularly for solids. This can be improved by acute intravenous or intramuscular injection of gastrokinetic drugs, but has not been confirmed in a larger double-blind trial using oral domperidone for 14 days. Hence, whereas individual patients may experience symptomatic relief, the use of gastrokinetic drugs as an adjunct in the overall management of low-weight anorexic patients is not recommended at present but rather needs further exploration.

REFERENCES

Bennett, H.P.J., & McMartin, C. Peptide hormones and their analogues: Distribution, clearance from the circulation and inactivation in vivo. *Pharmacological Rev.*, 30:247–292, 1978.

Brener, W., Hendrix, T. R., & McHugh, P. R. Regulation of the gastric emptying of glucose. *Gastroenterol.,* 85:76–82, 1983.

Brogden, R. N., Carmine, A. A., Heel, R. C., Speight, T. M., & Avery, G. S. Domperidone: A review of its pharmacological activity, pharmacokinetics and therapeutic efficacy in the symptomatic treatment of chronic dyspepsia and as an antiemetic. *Drugs,* 24:360–400, 1982.

Cannon, W. B. The movement of the stomach studied by the means of roentgen rays. *Am. J. Physiol.,* 1:359–382, 1898.

Cannon, W. B., & Washburn, A. L. An explanation of hunger. *Am. J. Physiol.,* 29:441–445, 1912.

Coates, G., Gilday, D. L., Cradduck, T. D., & Wood, D. E. Measurement of the rate of stomach emptying using Indium 113n and a 10 crystal rectilinear scanner. *Can. Med. Assoc. J.,* 115:180–183, 1973.

Costall, B., Gunning, S. J., Naylor, R. J., & Simpson, K. H. A central site of action for benzamide facilitation of gastric emptying. *Eur. J. Pharmacol.,* 91:197–205, 1983.

Dixon, K., Zip, F. W., O'Dorisio, T., & Cataland, S. Release of gastric inhibitory polypeptide (GIP) in anorexia nervosa pretreatment and during weight recovery. Abstract. Presented at International Symposium on Disorders of Eating, Pavia, Italy, 1985.

Dixon, K., Zip, F. W., O'Dorisio, T., & Cataland, S. In E. Ferrari (Ed.), *Advances in Bioscience.* New York: Pergamon Press, in press.

Dubois, A., Gross, H. A., Ebert, M. H., & Castell, D. O. Altered gastric emptying and secretion in primary anorexia nervosa. *Gastroenterol.,* 77:319–323, 1979.

Dubois, A., Gross, H. A., Richter, J. E., & Ebert, M. H. Effect of bethanechol on gastric function in primary anorexia nervosa. *Dig. Dis. & Sci.,* 26:598–600, 1981.

Edin, R., Lundberg, J., Terenius, L., Dahlstrom, D., Hokfelt, J., Kewenter, J., & Dhleman, H. Evidence for vagal encephalinergic neural control of feline pylorus and stomach. *Gastroenterol.,* 78:492–497, 1980.

Euler, A. R. Use of bethanecol for the treatment of gastroesophageal reflux. *J. Pediatr.,* 96:321–324, 1980.

Evans, D. S. Acute dilatation and spontaneous rupture of the stomach. *Br. J. Surg.,* 55:940–942, 1968.

Garfinkel, P. E., Moldofsky, H., & Garner, D. M. The stability of perceptual disturbances in anorexia nervosa. *Psychol. Med.,* 9:703–708, 1978.

Garfinkel, P. E., & Coscina, D. V. The physiology and psychology of hunger and satiety. In M. Zales (Ed.), *Eating, Sleeping and Sexuality.* New York: Brunner/Mazel, 1982.

Grill, B. B., Hilemeier, A. C., Semeraro, L. A., McCallum, R. W., & Gryboski, J. D. Effects of domperidone therapy on symptoms and upper gastrointestinal motility in infants with gastroesophageal reflux. *J. Pediatr.,* 106:311-316, 1985.

Grimes, J. D., Hassan, M. N., & Preston, D. N. Adverse neurologic effects of metoclopramide. *Can. Med. Assoc. J.,* 126:23-25, 1982.

Guyton, A. C. *Textbook of Medical Physiology* (5th ed.). Philadelphia: W. B. Saunders, 1986, pp. 691, 764, 765.

Heykants, J., Hendriks, R., Meuldermaus, W., Michiels, M., Scheygroud, H., & Reyntjeus, H. On the pharmacokinetics of domperidone in animals and man. *Eur. J. Drug Metabol. Pharmacokinetics,* 6:61-70, 1981.

Hitch, D. C., Vanhoutte, J. J., & Torres-Pinedo, R. B. Enhanced gastroduodenal motility in children. *Am. J. Dis. Child.,* 136:299, 1982.

Holt, S., Ford, M. J., Grant, S., & Heading, R. C. Abnormal gastric emptying in primary anorexia nervosa. *Br. J. Psychiatry,* 139:550-552, 1981.

Hunt, J. N., & Spurrell, W. P. The pattern of emptying of the human stomach. *J. Physiol.,* 113:157-168, 1951.

Hunt, J. N., & Know, M. T. The slowing of gastric emptying by four strong acids and three weak acids. *J. Physiol.,* 222:187-208, 1972.

Lundberg, J. M., Horfelt, T., Kewenter, J., Petterson, G., Ahlman, H., Edin, R., Dahlstrom, A., Nilsson, G., Teremus, L., Uvmas-Nallensten, K., & Said, S. Substance P, VIP and enkephalin like immunoreactivity in the human vagus nerve. *Gastroenterol.,* 77:468-471, 1979.

McCallum, R. W., Fink, S. M., Lerner, E., & Berkowitz, D. M. Effects of metoclopramide and bethanecol on delayed gastric emptying present in gastroesophageal reflux patients. *Gastroenterol.,* 84:1573-1577, 1983.

McCallum, R. W., Grill, B. B., Lange, R., Planky, M., Glass, E. E., & Greenfield, D. G. Definition of a gastric emptying abnormality in patients with anorexia nervosa. *Dig. Dis. Sci.* (new series), 30(8), 1985.

McHugh, P. R., & Moran, J. H. The stomach: A conception of its dynamic role in satiety. In J. Sprague & A. Epstein (Eds.), *Progress in Psychobiology and Physiological Psychology,* vol. II. New York: Academic Press, 1985.

Meyer, J. H., Ohashi, H., Jehn, D., & Thompson, J. B. Size of liver particles emptied from the human stomach. *Gastroenterol.*, 80:1489-1496, 1981.

Minami, H., & McCallum, R. W. The physiology and pathophysiology of gastric emptying in humans. *Gastroenterol.*, 86:1592-1610, 1984.

Moldofsky, H., Jeuniewic, N., & Garfinkel, P. E. Preliminary report on metoclopramide in anorexia nervosa. In R. A. Vigersky (Ed.), *Anorexia Nervosa.* New York: Raven Press, 1977, pp. 373-375.

Nelson, J. D., & Solyom, L. Response of the hormones of the gastro-entero-pancreatic axis to a test meal in anorexia nervosa, bulimia, and normal controls (Abstract). Presented at International Symposium on Disorders of Eating Behaviour, Pavia, Italy, 1985.

Ross, G. (Ed.). *Essentials of Human Physiology.* Chicago: Yearbook Publishers, 1978, pp. 388, 391.

Russell, D. McR., Freedman, M. L., Feiglin, D.H.I., Jeejeebhoy, K. N., Swinson, R. P., & Garfinkel, P. E. Delayed gastric emptying and improvement with domperidone in a patient with anorexia nervosa. *Am. J. Psychiatry,* 140:1235-1236, 1983.

Russell, G.F.M. Acute dilatation of the stomach in a patient with anorexia nervosa. *Br. J. Psychiatry,* 112:203-207, 1966.

Saleh, J. W., & Lebwohl, P. Metoclopramide induced gastric emptying in patients with anorexia nervosa. *Am. J. Gastroenterol.,* 74:127-132, 1980.

Schuurkes, J.A.J., & Van Nueten, J. M. Control of gastroduodenal coordination: Dopaminergic and cholinergic pathways. *Scand. J. Gastroenter.* (Suppl B), 92:8-12, 1984.

Scobie, B. A. Acute gastric dilatation and duodenal ileus in anorexia nervosa. *Med. J. Australia,* ii:932-934, 1973.

Silverstone, J. T., & Russell, G.F.M. Gastric 'hunger' contractions in anorexia nervosa. *Br. J. Psychiatry,* 113:257-263, 1967.

Stacher, G., Bergmann, H., Wiesnagrotzki, S., Kiss, A., Hobarth, J., & Mittelbach, G. Anorexia nervosa and bulimia: Delayed gastric emptying accelerated by cisapride (Abstract). Presented at International Symposium on Disorders of Eating Behaviour, Pavia, Italy, 1985a.

Stacher, G., Kiss, A., Wiesnagrotzki, S., Bergmann, H., Havlik, E., & Mittlebach, G. Abnormal esophageal motility and gastric emptying in patients diagnosed as having primary anorexia nervosa. Abstract.

Presented at International Symposium on Disorders of Eating Behaviour, Pavia, Italy, 1985b.

Strunz, U. T., & Grossman, M. T. Electrointragastric pressure on gastric emptying and secretion. *Am. J. Physiol.,* 235:E552–555, 1978.

Thomas, P. A., Kelly, K. A., & Go, V.L.W. Does motilin regulate canine interdigestive motility. *Dig. Dis. Sci.,* 24:577–582, 1979.

Track, N. S. The gastrointestinal endocrine system. *Can. Med. Assoc. J.,* 122:287–292, 1980.

Valenzuela, J. E. Dopamine as a possible neurotransmitter in gastric relaxations. *Gastroenterol.,* 71:1019–1022, 1976.

Wallin, L., Madsen, T., & Boesby, S. Effect of domperidone on gastroesophageal function in normal human subjects. *Scand. J. Gastroenter.,* 20:150–154, 1985.

Wiholm, B. E., Mortimer, O., Boethius, G., & Haggstrom, J. E. Tardive dyskinesia associated with metoclopramide. *Br. Med. J.,* 288:545–547, 1984.

Wilbur, B., & Kelly, R. Effect of proximal gastric, complete gastric and truncal vagotomy on canine gastric electrical activity, motility, and emptying. *Ann. Surg.,* 178:295–300, 1973.

Name Index

Abdec-Fatiah, M.H., 150, 153
Abraham, S.F., 5
Albala, A.A., 7
Allers, G., 78
Anand, B.K., 98, 125, 136
Ananth, J., 76
Andersen, A.E., 59-60, 64
Andersen, R.N., 150
Anderson, G.H., 96, 126-128, 138
Annable, L., 138
Antelman, S.M., 142
Ashcroft, G.W., 138
Atkinson, R.L., 151, 156
Avery, G., 169

Badawy, A.A., 108, 130
Ballenger, J., 14-15, 110, 130
Bansal, S., 137
Baranowska, B., 150, 153
Barchas, J., 125
Barratt, K.H., 47
Barry, V.C., 74, 80
Bartlett, D., 15, 24
Battacharya, G., 94
Beitman, B.D., 76
Bellin, B., 99
Ben David, M., 82
Benady, D.R., 132
Bennett, H.P.J., 165
Berchou, R., 14
Bergen, S.S., 132
Bergmann, H., 168, 170
Berkowitz, D.M., 169
Berrettini, W.H., 150
Beumont, P.J.V., 5
Bhanji, S., 76
Bhatnager, O.P., 136
Bialos, D., 11
Biederman, J., 4, 6, 21, 38, 40
Billington, C.J., 152
Bjorkquist, S.E., 111
Blavet, N., 136

Blinder, B.J., 78
Bloom, R.E., 151
Blumberg, A.G., 94
Blundell, J.E., 125-126, 139
Boethius, G., 170
Boyar, R.M., 8
Brainard, J., 141
Brands, B., 151, 156
Bray, G.A., 107
Brener, W., 162
Brinkley, J.R., 76
Brobeck, J.R., 125
Brock, J.T., 110
Brogden, R.N., 169
Brotman, A.W., 45
Brown, G.L., 130
Brown, G.M., 96, 114
Brown, W.A., 137
Brownstein, M.J., 152
Brozek, J., 10
Bruch, H., 4, 62, 75
Buchsbaum, M.S., 26
Burdizk, E.G., 11
Burroughs, J., 4, 6, 37, 38, 52, 96, 130
Burrow, G.N., 126-127
Busch, A.K., 100
Byerley, B., 141
Byerley, W.F., 137
Bymaster, F.P., 141

Cade, J.F.J., 90
Caille, G., 92
Calabrese, J., 8
Campbell, I.C., 15-16, 23
Campus, P.E., 100
Candy, J., 14
Cannon, W.B., 162
Cantwell, D.P., 4, 6, 37, 52, 96
Carmine, A.A., 169
Carrillo, C., 94
Carroll, B.J., 7
Casper, R., 4

Castell, D.O., 167
Cataland, S., 165, 168
Cereghino, J.J., 110
Chakrabarty, A.S., 136
Chakrabarty, K., 136
Charney, D.S., 92
Checkley, S.A., 126, 140
Chiles, J.A., 100
Chmara, J., 75
Chouinard, G.C., 138, 141
Chrousos, G.P., 8
Clostre, F., 136
Coates, G., 171
Coble, P., 9
Cohen, D.J., 129
Cohen, J., 21, 135
Cohen, M.R., 151, 156, 158
Cohen, R.M., 15-16, 23, 26, 151, 156, 158
Cohen, S., 71
Conroy, R., 81-82
Cooper, P.J., 5, 6
Coscina, D.V., 99, 164
Costall, B., 166
Cournoyer, G., 92
Cowdry, R.W., 109
Cradduck, T.D., 171
Craigen, G., 161-176
Crawford, T.B.B., 138
Crisp, A.H., 40, 43, 61-62, 75, 78-77, 97
Cunningham, C.J., 46

Dacaney, E.P., 131
Dahlstrom, D., 166
Dahms, W.T., 107
Dalby, M., 97, 109
Dalle Ore, G., 99
Dally, P.J., 15, 77-79, 82
Damiouji, N.F., 44
Dan, V., 82
Daneman, D., 115
Darby, P.L., 111
Davidson, J., 11, 20
Davis, J., 4, 15
Davis, K.L., 102, 106-107, 114
Davis, L., 92
DeCastro, R.M., 137
DeFeudis, F.V., 136
DeMontigny, C., 92
Dermer, S.W., 101, 109
Desbuquois, G., 82
DeSouza, V., 4
Dettman, P.W., 151, 156
Dibble, E.D., 6, 37
Dijken, W.A., 18
Dixon, K.N., 7, 9, 38, 165, 168

Doerr, P., 98
Doran, A.R., 151, 156
Dubois, A., 167, 169-170
Dufay, F., 78
Duncan, W., 9
Duw, S., 98
Dyrenfurth, I., 8

Ebert, M.H., 5, 37, 91, 93, 129, 150, 153-154, 167, 169-170
Eccleston, D., 138
Eckert, E., 4, 6, 21, 37, 40, 134, 135
Edelstein, C.K., 43
Edin, R., 166
Engel, K., 79
Euler, A.R., 168
Evans, D.S., 161
Evans, M., 108, 130

Faden, V.B., 91, 93
Fairbanks, L., 129
Fairburn, C.G., 5, 6
Falk, J.R., 37, 40, 135
Farnum, C., 102
Farquhar, D.L., 139
Farrington, A.J., 47
Feighenbaum, Z.S., 102
Feiglin, D.H.I., 171
Feinberg, M., 7
Fenton, G.W., 97
Ferber, R.A., 4, 21, 38
Ferguson, J.M., 44, 126, 142
Fichter, M., 98
Fingeroth, S., 9
Fink, S.M., 169
Folstein, M.F., 4
Fontaine, R., 45-46
Ford, M.J., 167
Foster, F.G., 9, 97
Frahm, H., 78-79
Frankel, B.L., 9
Freedman, M.L., 171
Freeman, C., 142
Freeman, D.M.A., 78
Freeman, R.J., 76
Frenk, J., 151, 156
Friedel, R.O., 76
Frommer, E., 14
Fuchs, C.Z., 11, 14
Fukushima, D., 7
Fuller, R.W., 126, 141

Gallagher, T.F., 7
Galloway, S.M., 139
Gardner, D.L., 109

Name Index

Gardner, M., 14, 24
Garfinkel, P.E., 4–6, 8, 19, 24–26, 79, 96, 99, 111, 114–115, 126–127, 130, 135–136, 161, 164, 170–171
Garner, D.M., 79, 96, 111, 130, 135–136, 161
Garner, R.H., 43
Garrick, N., 15–16, 23, 26
George, T., 150
Gerner, R.H., 8, 38, 96, 129, 153–154
Gershon, E.S., 6, 37
Ghafoor, P.K.A., 78
Gibbs, E.L., 101–102
Gibbs, F.A., 101–102
Gilday, D.L., 171
Gillberg, C., 129
Giller, E., 11
Gillin, J.C., 9
Gillman, M.A., 94, 155
Gittelman, E.R., 10, 23
Givens, J.R., 150
Gladis, M., 5, 8, 18–19, 22, 24, 26, 37
Glass, E.E., 167, 169–170
Glassman, A.H., 5, 8–9, 18–19, 22, 24, 26, 37
Glick, B.S., 11
Glover, V., 26
Go, V.L.W., 166
Goetz, R.R., 9
Goff, G., 92
Gold, P.W., 8, 150
Goldberg, S.C., 4, 91, 93, 134
Goldbloom, D.S., 124–143
Gomez de Martin Borado, H., 82–83
Gomez, J., 78–79, 82
Goodwin, D.W., 130
Goodwin, F.K., 27, 130
Goor, E., 97
Gosnell, B.A., 152
Goudie, A.J., 126, 141
Gowdey, C.W., 151, 156
Grace, W.J., 100
Gram, L.F., 94
Grant, S., 167
Grebb, J.A., 97
Greden, J.F., 7
Green, J.K., 4, 6, 96
Green, R.S., 100–103, 106
Greenfield, D.G., 167, 169–170
Greenway, F.L., 107
Grill, B.B., 167, 169–170
Grimes, J.D., 170
Groat, R.A., 47
Grochochinski, V., 9
Groh, C., 109

Gross, H.A., 91, 93, 167, 169–170
Gross, M., 79
Grosser, B.I., 141
Grossman, A., 153
Grossman, M.T., 164
Grossman, S.P., 126
Grounds, A., 75
Gryboski, J.D., 169
Guirguis, W., 14
Gunning, S.J., 166
Guyton, A.C., 162, 166
Gwirtsman, H.E., 8, 38, 43, 96, 129, 150

Haggstrom, J.E., 170
Halmi, K.A., 4, 21, 37, 40, 78–79, 134, 135
Halpern, F.S., 7
Hamilton, D., 6
Hamilton, M., 15
Hamovit, J.R., 6, 37
Hanaoka, M., 110
Harmatz, J.S., 6, 21, 38
Harper, G.P., 4, 6, 21, 38, 40
Harrison, W., 15, 18, 22
Hartshorn, J., 91, 93
Hassan, M.N., 170
Hatsukami, D., 37
Havlik, E., 168
Hazama, H., 111
Heading, R.C., 167
Heel, R.C., 169
Hellman, L.D., 7–8
Hendren, R.L., 37
Hendrix, T.R., 162
Heninger, G.R., 92
Henschel, A., 10
Herishanu, Y., 99
Hernandez-Peon, R., 108
Herridae, P.L., 45–46
Herz, A., 153
Herzog, D.B., 4–6, 21, 36–38, 40, 45
Heseltine, G.F.D., 14
Hessbacher, P., 126
Hetherington, A.W., 98
Heykants, J., 173
Hilemeier, A.C., 169
Himmelhoch, J.M., 11, 14
Hirst, M., 151, 156
Hitch, D.C., 169
Hobarth, J., 168, 170
Hoebel, B.G., 126
Hoes, M.J.A., 81
Hofstatter, L., 100
Hollister, L.E., 102, 106–107, 114, 117
Holt, S., 167
Hooshmand, H., 111

Horfelt, T., 166
Horne, R., 44
Horng, J.S., 141
Hosfiel, W., 102
Houseworth, S., 6, 38
Howard, D., 15
Hrboticky, N., 126–127, 138
Hsu, L.K.G., 4, 60, 75, 90–94
Hudson, J.I., 5–6, 8–9, 21, 24–25, 37–39, 43, 45–46, 75, 96, 106, 115
Hudson, M.S., 115
Hughes, P.C., 46
Hunt, J.N., 162
Huttgren, H., 93
Hytell, J., 131

Inanago, S., 110
Inoue, H., 110
Inoue, K., 111
Isohanni, B., 111
Ives, J.O., 15, 24

Jacobs, C., 38
Jacobsen, G., 14–15
Jeejeebhoy, K.N., 171
Jenn, D., 164
Jeske, W., 150, 153
Jeuniewic, N., 170
Jimerson, D.C., 150
Joffe, R.T., 111
Johnson, C., 5, 115
Johnson, J.P., 26
Johnson, L., 115
Johnson-Sabine, E., 47
Johnston, J.L., 126–127, 128
Jonas, J.M., 5–6, 8–9, 21, 24–25, 37–39, 43, 45, 75, 96
Jones, J., 91, 93
Jones, M.W., 100

Kaffman, M., 75
Kamp, J.S., 18
Kao, J., 93
Kaplan, A.S., 96, 111, 114, 130
Karoum, F., 26
Katz, J., 8–9
Kay, D., 109
Kaye, W.H., 6, 91, 93, 129, 150, 153–154
Kayser, A., 15
Kellner, C.H., 8
Kelly, D., 14
Kelly, K.A., 166
Kelly, R., 167
Kemper, K., 6, 38
Kennedy, S., 4–6, 8, 19, 24–26, 96

Kenshole, A., 115
Kewenter, J., 166
Keys, A., 10
Khanna, J.L., 11
Kirschbaum, W.R., 99–100
Kishimoto, A., 110–111
Kiss, A., 168, 170
Kitabchi, A.E., 150
Klawans, H.L., 74, 80
Klein, D.F., 10, 15, 23, 94
Know, M.T., 162
Kocan, D., 142
Kopanda, P.P., 108
Kosterlitz, H.W., 152
Krahn, D., 138
Krieger, D.T., 152
Kruzik, P., 126
Kuhn, R., 78, 109
Kunzer, W., 79
Kuperberg, A., 9
Kupfer, D.J., 9

Lacey, J.H., 40, 43
Lacy, W.W., 133
LaDu, T.J., 21, 135
Lafeber, C., 78
Laffer, P.S., 37
Lake, C.R., 129
Lake, M.D., 7, 38
Lamborn, J., 14, 24
Lange, R., 167, 169–170
Langlois, R., 92
Lantz, S., 7
Larkin, C., 81–82
Larsen, J.J., 131
Larson, R., 5, 115
Lasagna, L., 131
Latham, C.J., 126, 139
Lavenstein, A.F., 131
Lawrin, M.O., 131
Lebwohl, P., 168–169
Lee, L.E., 91, 93
Leiter, L.A., 126–127, 138
Lerner, E., 169
Lesham, M.B., 126, 139
Levine, A.S., 125, 150, 152
Levitz, L., 106
Levy, A.B., 9
Lewidge, B., 14
Lewis, M.J., 150
Li, E.T.S., 126–127
Lichtigfeld, E.J., 94, 155
Liddle, G.W., 133
Liebowitz, M.R., 15
Liebowitz, S.F., 139

Name Index

Lindy, D.C., 8
Lingao, A., 100
Linnoila, M., 11, 26–27
Liotta, A.S., 152
Lipper, S., 26
Loriaux, D.L., 134
Luby, E., 155
Luciano, M., 151, 156
Ludden, C.T., 131
Lund, R., 98
Lundberg, J., 166
Lundberg, O., 97
Lynn, A.G., 151, 156

MacFayden, J., 6
Major, L.F., 130
Makela, R., 111
Malinen, L., 111
March, V., 6, 38, 96
Marchelli, E.A., 82–83
Margules, D.L., 150
Mark, S., 140
Markowitz, J.S., 15
Martin, A., 83
Masson, J.M., 83
Masterson, J.F., 76
Matsumoto, H., 110
McCallum, R.W., 167, 169–170
McCarthy, P.S., 151, 156
McClure, D.J., 14
McGrath, P.J., 18
McHugh, P.R., 162, 164–165
McKenna, P.J., 75
McMartin, C., 165
Meermann, R., 80, 84, 96
Meltzer, E.S., 75
Mendels, J., 6, 38, 43, 96
Mendis, N., 26
Merlkangus, J.R., 97
Meyer, A.E., 79
Meyer, J.H., 164
Mickalide, A.D., 64
Mickelsen, O., 10
Miles, J.E., 76
Mills, I.H., 150, 154–155, 157
Mitchell, J., 6, 37, 47, 92, 102, 138
Mitchell-Heggs, N., 14
Mittelbach, G., 168, 170
Moisset, B., 150
Moldofsky, H., 130, 161, 170
Molloy, B.B., 126, 141
Moore, D.C., 39
Moore, R., 150, 154–155, 157
Moore, S.L., 106
Moran, J.H., 164–165

Morissette, R., 92
Morley, J.E., 125, 150, 152–153
Morrell, W., 6, 38, 130
Mortimer, O., 170
Morton, R., 59
Moses, P.L., 127, 137
Moskovitz, R.A., 100
Munford, P.R., 83
Munro, A., 75
Munro, J.F., 139
Murphy, D.L., 15–16, 23, 26–27, 151, 156, 158
Mystener, A., 110

Naber, D., 150, 153–154
Nakamura, T., 136
Naranjo, C.A., 131
Nasrallah, H.A., 9
Naylor, G., 109
Naylor, R.J., 166
Needleman, H.L., 39
Nell, J.F., 97
Nelson, J.D., 168
Nemzer, E., 7, 38
Niang, I., 82
Niederhoff, H., 79
Nies, A., 14–15, 24
Noble, R.E., 132
Nolan, W.A., 18

O'Dorisio, T., 165, 168
Obura, C., 111
Ohashi, H., 164
Okuma, T., 110
Ono, T., 136
Oomura, Y., 136
Oppenheim, G.B., 77
Orxulak, P.J. (Biederman), 21
Otsuki, K., 110
Owens, M., 4–6, 96

Pare, C.M.B., 10, 21, 26
Parker, R.R., 15
Parsons, J.M., 98
Paterson, S.J., 152
Paupe, J., 82
Paykel, E.S., 15
Penny, J.K., 110
Perry, K.W., 126, 141
Pert, C.B., 150–151, 156
Petterson, G., 166
Pettigrew, K.D., 9
Pfeiffer, A., 153
Pickar, D., 150–151, 153–154, 156, 158

Piennes, M.G., 83
Pierloot, R., 81–82
Pillai, R.V., 136
Piran, N., 4–6, 8, 19, 24–26, 96
Pirke, K.M., 98
Planky, M., 167, 169–170
Plantey, F., 81
Plum, F., 99
Pohl, R., 14
Pollack, C.P., 9
Pope, H.G., 5–6, 8–9, 21, 24–25, 37–39, 43, 45–46, 75, 96, 106
Post, R.M., 8, 108, 110–111
Potter, W.Z., 27
Pratt, S., 11
Preston, D.N., 170
Puente, R.M., 109
Pyle, R., 6, 37, 102

Quallis, B., 106
Quitkin, F., 10, 15, 18, 22, 23, 94

Rabkin, J., 15, 22
Rafaelson, O.J., 94
Rainey, J.M., 14
Rakes, S.M., 106
Raleigh, M., 129
Ranson, S., 98
Rau, J.H., 100–103, 106
Ravaris, C.L., 15, 24
Ravindranath, 78
Recant, L., 151, 156
Reeves, A.G., 99
Reid, A., 109
Reimherr, F.W., 141
Remick, R.A., 100
Remschmidt, H., 110
Reus, V.I., 97
Reynolds, E.H., 108
Rich, C.L., 18, 25
Richter, J.E., 169–170
Rickels, J., 126
Riddle, M., 11
Riederen, P., 126
Rifkin, A., 10, 23, 94
Risch, S.C., 137
Rivinus, T.M., 4, 6, 21, 38, 40
Roberts, F.J., 77
Robinson, D.S., 14, 15, 24
Robinson, P.H., 126, 140
Robson, L.E., 152
Rodin, G., 115
Roffwarg, H.P., 7, 8
Rogers, G.H., 151, 156
Roig, M., 37

Roose, S.P., 5, 8–9, 18–19, 22, 24, 26, 37
Rose, S., 24
Rosenbaum, J.F., 21
Rosenberg, P., 99
Ross, C.A., 131
Ross, G., 164–165
Rossignol, C., 82
Rouger, M.E., 83
Rowan, P.R., 15
Rowland, N., 142
Roy, A., 8
Roy, B., 26
Roy-Byrne, P., 8, 43, 96, 111
Rozbicka, G., 150, 153
Russell, D., 171
Russell, G.F.M., 5, 62, 115, 126, 140, 161, 167

Sachar, E.J., 7
Sadik, C., 5, 37
Saleh, J.W., 168, 169
Salicia, B., 38
Salkin, B., 4, 6, 96, 130
Sandler, M., 26
Sanger, D.J., 150–151, 156
Sansone, R.A., 7
Sapse, A.T., 98
Sarai, R., 110
Sargant, W., 14, 15, 77
Schildkraut, J.J. (Biederman), 21
Schmidt, H.A., 9
Schnaultz, N.L., 39
Schreiber, J.L., 6, 37
Schrier, S.S., 7
Schroeder, J.S., 93
Schuurkes, J.A.J., 169
Schuyler, D., 133
Scobie, B.A., 167
Scotton, L., 97
Sellers, E.M., 131
Selvini Palazzoli, M., 75
Semeraro, L.A., 169
Sepdham, T., 111
Sharp, B., 153–154
Sheehan, D.V., 14–15
Shibuya, H., 150
Sholomskas, A., 11
Siever, L.J., 15–16, 23, 26
Silverstone, J.T., 133, 167
Simpson, K.H., 166
Singh, B., 136
Slater, S., 26
Smeltzer, D.J., 7
Smith, L.D., 110
Smolik, E.A., 100

Name Index

Snyder, F., 9
Solyom, C., 14
Solyom, L., 14, 76, 168
Sours, J., 79
Sovner, R., 137
Speight, T.M., 169
Spitzer, R.L., 15
Stacher, G., 168, 170
Stark, P., 141
Stavorski, J.M., 131
Stein, G.S., 91, 93
Steinberg, D., 14, 91, 93
Stern, G.M., 26
Stern, S.L., 7, 38
Stern-Mighton, D., 8
Sternberg, D.E., 92
Stewart, J.W., 15, 18-19, 22, 24, 26, 96
Stiel, J.N., 133
Stokl, S., 8
Stone, C.A., 131
Stricker, E.M., 94
Strober, M., 4, 6, 38, 130
Strunz, U.T., 164
Struve, F.A., 101-102
Stunkard, A.J., 78, 100, 102, 106-107, 114, 126
Sturzenberger, S., 4, 6, 37, 52, 96
Sugimori, M., 136
Sullivan, J., 11
Sunderland, T., 23
Swinson, R.P., 171
Symons, B.J., 11, 14
Szmukler, G.I., 115, 130

Takezoki, H., 110
Tantam, D., 130
Tarika, J., 7
Taylor, H.L., 10
Terenius, L., 166
Terzian, A., 99
Theander, S., 4, 6
Thomas, C.D., 76
Thomas, C.S., 75
Thomas, P.A., 166
Thompson, J.B., 164
Thorhill, J.A., 151, 156
Thornton, E.W., 126, 141
Thouvenot, J., 83
Tilkian, A.G., 93
Toifl, K., 126
Torres-Pinedo, R.B., 169
Toudorf, R., 21
Track, N.S., 166
Trainor, D., 75
Tricamo, E., 15, 22

Trulson, M.E., 127
Tryon, W.W., 135
Tunks, E.R., 101, 109
Turnbull, C., 11, 20
Tyano, S., 82
Tyrer, P., 14, 24

Uhde, T.W., 111
Usdin, E., 125

Valenzuela, J.E., 166
Van de Putten, J.J., 18
Van Metre, T.E., 131
Van Nueten, J.M., 169
Van Praag, H.M., 125
Vande Wiele, R., 8
Vandereycken, W., 80, 81-84
Vanhoutte, J.J., 169
VanMeter, J.C., 110
Vaucheret, G., 82-83
Vialatte, J., 82
Viesselman, J.O., 37
Vigersky, R.A., 134
Vittouris, N., 78
Volmat, R., 78
Voyles, N.R., 151, 156
Vries, J.K., 111

Waber, D., 39
Wakeling, A., 4, 47
Walinder, J., 97
Walsh, B.T., 5, 8-9, 18-19, 22, 24, 26, 37, 96
Walsh, N., 81-82
Warsh, J.J., 96, 114, 128
Washburn, A.L., 162
Wegner, J.R., 101
Wehr, T.A., 27
Weingartner, H., 158
Weiss, J., 11
Weiss, S.R., 5, 37, 129
Weiss, T., 106
Weizman, R., 82
Wells, C.A., 46
Wenger, H.C., 131
Wentworth, S.M., 115
Wermuth, B.M., 102, 106-107, 114
West, E.D., 15
Wheeler, T.J., 126, 141
White, B.G., 110
White, J.H., 39
Whitford, M., 14, 24
Whittier, J.R., 99
Wiedmann, E., 150
Wiesler, B., 79

Wiesnagrotzki, S., 168, 170
Wiholm, B.E., 170
Wijsenbeek, H., 82
Wilbur, B., 167
Wilkes, B., 8
Wilkus, R.J., 100
Williams, J.B.W., 15
Winokur, A., 6, 38, 96
Wise, T.N., 151, 156
Wolff, H.G., 100
Wolkowitz, O.M., 151, 156
Wong, D.T., 141-142
Wood, D.E., 171
Wood, D.R., 141
Woods, S.W., 45
Wright, L., 8, 96
Wu, P.H., 131
Wurtman, J.J., 127, 137, 140-141

Wurtman, R.J., 127, 137, 140-141
Wyatt, R.J., 26

Yager, J., 8, 43, 96
Yen, T.T., 142
Yingling, C.D., 97
Yonace, A., 47
Young, S.N., 137, 138
Yurgelun-Todd, D., 5-6, 21, 25, 37-39, 45-46, 96

Zarr, M.L., 76
Zimmerman, E.A., 152
Zip, F.W., 165, 168
Zisook, S., 11
Zukin, R.S., 152
Zukin, S.R., 152
Zumoff, B., 8, 9

Subject Index

Acetyl transferase, 23–24
Acidic solutions, 162
Adrenocorticotrophin hormone (ACTH), 152, 166
Affective disorders
  carbamazepine and, 110–111
  eating disorders and, 3–10, 36–38
  fluoxetine and, 141
  monoamine oxidase inhibitors and, 11–14
  tryptophan and, 137
Agranulocytosis, 80
Alcoholism, 37, 67, 69
  carbamazepine and, 111
  hyposerotoninergic state and, 130–131
Alzheimer's disease, 99
Amenorrhea, 83
Amino acid intake, 99
Amitriptyline, 15, 21, 39–42, 45, 47, 141
  combined with perphenazine, 79
  naloxone and, 155
  seizure disorders and, 116
  side effects, 50, 53
  versus cyproheptadine, 135–136
Amphetamine, 127
Anemia, 51
Anorexia nervosa
  amphetamine-induced, 23
  anxiety and, 62–63
  cyproheptadine and, 133–137
  dopaminergic activity and, 74–75
  family history and, 6
  gastric emptying and, 167–168, 171–176
  gastrointestinal symptoms of, 161
  hypothalamic-pituitary-adrenal axis abnormalities, 7–8
  lithium and, 90–91
  medical complications of, 51
  monoamine oxidase inhibitors and, 20–21
  mood disturbances and, 3–10
  opioid antagonists and, 150, 154–158
  place of medication in treating, 54
  role of psychopharmacological agents in, 60–61
  similarities between alcoholism and, 130
  sleep disturbances and, 9–10
  tricyclic antidepressants and, 38–43, 49
Antianxiety agents, *see* Tranquilizers
Anticonvulsants, 96–117
Antrum, 164, 167–168
Anxiety, 5
  eating disorders and, 62–64
  monoamine oxidase inhibitors and, 14
Appetite
  drugs to increase, 60
  opioid peptides and, 151–153

Beck Depression Inventory, 92
Behavior therapy, 25, 47, 49, 84
  pimozide treatments and, 82
Benzamphetamine, 142
Benzodiazepines, 71–72
Beta-endorphin, 151–154
Beta-lipotropin, 152
Bethanecol, 168–170
Binge eating
  anxiety and, 63–64, 68–69
  fenfluramine and, 139–140
  fluoxetine and, 142
  seizure disorders and, 100
Biopsychosocial model, 96
Bipolar disorder, 90
  carbamazepine and, 110
Blood glucose, 99
Body image disturbance, 75
Borderline personality disorder, 20
  anorexia nervosa as a form of, 76
  carbamazepine and, 109
Bradycardia, 51
Brain diseases, 99–100
Bulimia nervosa
  anxiety and, 63–64
  carbamazepine and, 111–115

Bulimia nervosa *(continued)*
   fluoxetine and, 142–143
   hypothalamic-pituitary-adrenal activity
     and, 8–9
   lithium and, 91–92
   medical complications of, 52
   monoamine oxidase inhibitors and, 18–20,
     25–26
   mood disturbances and, 3–10
   panic disorder and, 5
   place of medication in treating, 54
   as a seizure disorder, 100–103
   sleep disturbances and, 9–10
   tricyclic antidepressants and, 42–49
Buproprion, 44–45
Butyrophenones, 74

Carbamazepine, 105, 108–115
Carbohydrate intake, 127, 130, 137–140, 142
Cardiac abnormalities, 93
Cardiac arrhythmias, 52
Catecholamines, 38, 99, 128
Cerebrospinal fluid, 128–129, 153–154
Chlorpheniramine, 131
Chlorpromazine, 60, 74, 77–78, 83, 110
   disadvantages of, 79–80
Cholecystokinin (CCK), 164–166, 168
Chyme, 162
Cisapride, 167–170
Clomipramine, 40–41, 43
Clorgyline, 26–27
Cognitive behavior therapy, 25, 66
   lithium as an adjunct to, 91–92, 94
Computerized tomography, 97
Control, fear of loss of, 63
Convulsions, 97
Corticotropin releasing factor (CRF), 8
Cortisol, 7–8
Cyproheptadine, 40, 60, 71, 129, 131–137

Dehydration, 51–52
Denial of illness, 91
Deprenyl, 26–27
Depression
   cortisol secretion and, 7
   eating disorders and, 37–38, 49
   eating disorders as variants of, 4–10
   lithium and, 92
   major, 37, 50
   metoclopramide and, 170
Desipramine, 42, 45–46, 50–51, 53
Dexamethasone, 7–9, 38
Diabetes mellitus, 115
Dilantin, 103, 106

Diphenylbutylpiperidines, 124
Diphenylhydantoin, 60–61
Diuretics, 93
Domperidone, 169–176
Dopamine, 74, 80, 99
   gastric emptying and, 166
   lithium's effects on, 94
Drug abuse, 53, 69, 101
Duodenal mucosa, 164
Duodenum, 162, 164
Dynorphins, 152
Dyscontrol syndrome, 109
Dysmorphophobia, 75

EAT-26 questionnaire, 21
Eating Attitudes Test, 19, 92
Eating disorders, *see* Anorexia nervosa;
   Bulimia nervosa
ECT, 11, 15
Edema, 22
EEG, 61
   abnormal in bulimic patients, 97, 101–103,
     116
Electrocardiogram, 51
Electrolyte disturbances, 51–52
Encephalitis, 99
Endorphin, 151–154
Enkephalins, 152, 166
Enterogastric Reflex, 162
Enterogastrone, 164
Epilepsy, 80, 82
   carbamazepine and, 109
   eating disorders and, 116–117
Episodic dyscontrol syndrome, 101
Esophageal motility disorder, 168

Failing, fear of, 63
Family therapy, 66
Fatness, fear of, 62
Feeding behavior
   fenfluramine and, 139–140
   fluoxetine and, 141–142
   opioid peptides and, 151–153
   serotonin and, 125–128
   tryptophan and, 137–138
Feighner's criteria for depression, 37
Fenfluramine, 126–127, 137, 139–141
Fluoxetine, 126–127, 141–143
Fluphenazine, 74
Frahm method, 79

Galactorrhea, 83, 175
Gastric emptying
   control of, 162–166

Subject Index

drugs that facilitate, 168–176
Gastric inhibitory peptide (GIP), 164–165, 168
Gastrin, 164
Glucoregulatory hormones, 153
Gonadotropin, 153
Gut hormonal feedback, 166

Hallucinations, 101
Haloperidol, 74, 76, 83
Hamilton scores, 47
Headaches, 93, 101
Hemolytic anemia, 80
Histrionic personality, 15
Hopkins Symptom Checklist, 91
Hunger, 126
Huntington's chorea, 99
5-Hydroxyindolacetic acid, 129–130
5-Hydroxytryptophan, 126, 137
Hyperactivity, 79, 83
  carbamazepine and, 110
Hypercortisolism, 98
Hyperkinesia, 110
Hyperphagia, 98–99
Hyperprolactinemia, 80, 82
Hypertensive crises, 10
Hypertensive reactions, 21–22
Hypocalcemia, 52
Hypoglycemia, 116
Hypokalemia, 51, 116
Hypokinesia, 110
Hypotension, 22, 51
Hypothalamic-pituitary-adrenal axis, 7–9
Hypothalamus, 98, 100, 111, 125–126, 136, 153
Hysteroid dysphoria, 15, 23

Imipramine, 11, 15, 22, 39, 42, 45–47, 50–51, 53
Indoleamines, 38, 108
Insomnia, 50
Insulin, 77, 94, 99
  carbohydrate intake and, 127
Intragastric pressure, 164
Intubation technique, 167, 170
Isocarboxazid, 11, 19–20, 26
Isoleucine, 127

Kleine-Levin syndrome, 100
Kleptomania, 101
Kluver-Bucy syndrome, 99

Large neutral amino acids, 127–129
Laxatives, 93

Lesions, brain, 98–99
Leucine, 127
Leukopenia, 51, 80
Limbic system, 108–109
Lipid stores, 99
Lipotropin, 152
Lithium, 54, 61, 90–94
Liver dysfunction, 80
Lobotomy, 100
Lorazepam, 65–69

Major depressive disorder, 37, 50
Maprotiline, 117
3-methoxy-4 hydroxy phenylglycol (MHPG), 38, 40
Metoclopramide, 166, 168–170
Mianserin, 42, 45, 47
Monoamine oxidase inhibitors, 10–27, 39, 43–45, 53–54
  A and B subtypes, 26–27
  eating disorders and, 18–21
  lithium and, 92
  monitoring, 23–24
  side effects of, 21–22
  versus placebo, 11–14
  versus tricyclic antidepressants, 15–18
Monoamines, control of food intake and, 128
Monoideism, 75
Monosymptomatic hypochondriacal psychosis, 75
Mood disturbance, lithium and, 94
Morphine, 152
Mu receptor system, 152

Naloxone, 153, 155–158
Naltrexone, 155–157
Nausea, 93–94
Neuroendocrine measures, 38
Neuroleptics, 74–84
Neurotransmitters, 61, 99, 151
  carbamazepine and, 108–109
Night eaters, 100
NIMH Diagnostic Interview Schedule, 37
Nomifensine, 45
Nontricyclic antidepressants, 117
Norepinephrine, 99
  inhibition of monoamine oxidase and, 22–23
Norfenfluramine, 139

Obsessive-compulsive neurosis, 76
Operant conditioning, 78
Opioid peptides, 151–153

Oral contraceptives, 100
Orthostatic hypotension, 23
Oxazepam, 65

Pancreas, 153
Panic disorder, 5, 66, 71
Paranoia, intrapsychic, 75
Paresis, 100
Pargyline, 23
Parkinson's disease, 99
Parkinsonian dyskinetic reactions, 80
Perceptual distortion, 63
Perfectionism, 63
Peristalsis, 166
Perphenazine, 79
Personality disorders, 69
Phenelzine, 11, 14-15, 18-19, 24, 26
   side effects of, 22
Phenothiazines, 61, 74, 76-80
   seizure disorders and, 116
Phenylalanine, 127
Phenylethylamine, 23
Phenytoin, 98, 103-108, 115, 117
Pimozide, 81-83
Pituitary gland, 153
Present State Examination, 5
Pro-opiomelanocortin (POMC), 152
Probenicid, 129
Protein intake, 99
Psychiatric Rating Scale, 91
Psychotherapy, 52, 59
   chlorpromazine as an adjunct to, 77
Psychotic behavior, 53
Pyloric sphincter, 164

Rage attacks, 101
Relapse rate, 91-92
Relaxation methods, 66-67
REM latency, 9
Renal compromise, 51
Research Diagnostic Criteria (RDC), 37
Rituals, 50-51
Role playing, 66-67

Satiety, 126, 139, 141-142, 161
   gastric distension and, 162, 164
Schizophrenia, 75
Scintiscanning technique, 167, 171
SCL-90, 5, 37
Secretin, 164
Seizure disorders, 100-103
Self-esteem, 63

Serotonin, 99
   carbamazepine and, 108-109
   eating disorders and, 128-131
   feeding behavior and, 125-128
   inhibition of monoamine oxidase and, 22-23
Sexual dysfunction, 22
Sleep disturbances, 7, 9-10
   side effects of MAOIs and, 22
Small intestine, 162
Somatostatin, 166
Stress, 166
Sturge-Weber's Syndrome, 116
Suicide, 4, 102
Sulpiride, 74, 82-83
Sympathetic nervous system, 166
Sympathomimetics, 21

Tardive dyskinesia, 170
Temporal lobe abnormalities, 101
Tetrahydrocannabinol, 60, 71
Therapeutic alliance, 53
Thioridazine, 74
Thioxanthene, 74
Thought stopping, 66-67
Thought substitution, 67
Thyrotrophin-releasing hormone, 166
Tranquilizers
   major, 74-84
   potential misuses of, 69-71
   practice guidelines for, 64-69, 72
Tranylcypromine, 10-11, 14, 18, 26
Trazodone, 39, 43-45, 116
Triazolam, 69
Tricyclic antidepressants
   anorexia nervosa and, 38-43, 49
   approach to using, 49-54
   bulimia nervosa and, 42-49
   lithium and, 92
   monoamine oxidase inhibitors and, 15-18
   nontricyclic, 117
   seizure disorders and, 116
Tryptophan, 108, 126-127, 137-139
   levels in anorexics, 128-129
Tyramine, 21-22
Tyrosine, 127

Vagus nerve, 166
Valine, 127
Ventromedial nucleus, 98-99

Zimelidine, 131